WITHDRAWN
FROM LIBRARY

BRITISH MEDICAL ASSOCIATION

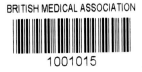

1001015

VANISHING BONE

ADVANCE PRAISE FOR *VANISHING BONE*

"Dr. William Harris, one of the seminal figures in joint replacement surgery, contributed to the improvement in health of countless people around the world. When the long-term benefits of that surgery were threatened by unforeseen complications, Dr. Harris and his colleagues embarked on understanding and restoring that benefit. This book documents that history and is a wonderful example of the contribution collaboration in science can make to people's health."

—SAMUEL O. THIER, MD, *Professor of Medicine and Health Care Policy, Emeritus, Harvard Medical School, Massachusetts General Hospital*

"At the crossroads of his leadership as both a clinician and research scientist lies the fascinating journey of discovery captured vividly in *Vanishing Bone*. A remarkably engaging read, the forty-year arc told by Dr. Harris is, at its heart, a wonderful mystery story. The relentless energy and dedication of Dr. Harris and his talented collaborators illustrate the promise of medical innovations that have benefited our families and millions around the world."

—JON ABBOTT, *President and CEO, WGBH, Boston-based TV and radio station*

"Hip replacement—called the "operation of the century"—was transforming the lives of millions of people, for the first time providing a cure for a crippling disease: hip arthritis. Just as the operation became popular, a surprising and unexpected problem developed that threatened its success: severe bone loss around the implants. The author of *Vanishing Bone* is an orthopaedic surgeon central to the development of the operation, and this is his personal story of the quest to understand and eventually find a solution to the problem. Dr. Harris skillfully traces this modern medical mystery and triumph—from recognition, to understanding, and finally to successful prevention—with captivating, true patient stories and an inside look at modern surgical practice and development of medical technology."

—DANIEL J. BERRY, MD, *L.Z. Gund Professor of Orthopaedic Surgery, Mayo Clinic*

"Periprosthetic osteolysis, bone destruction in the area of the prosthesis, was the silent killer of the fabulous expectations of total hip arthroplasty. Follow along as Dr. William Harris and his colleagues embark on a two-decade-long journey to eliminate this problem. You will explore the trials and tribulations these pioneers battled, along with the setbacks and restrictions of scientific discovery. Crosslinked polyethylene has revolutionized the field of total hip arthroplasty, permitting surgeons, in many cases, to give patients care that may last a lifetime. *Vanishing Bone* is a fascinating read."

—HARRY E. RUBASH, MD, *Chief Emeritus, Orthopaedic Surgery, Massachusetts General Hospital, Edith M. Ashley Professor of Orthopaedics, Harvard Medical School*

"Dr. Harris captures the science, the brilliance, the perseverance, and the serendipity that are involved in solving the world's most difficult medical problems. This book would be excellent for any curious reader as its mystery-like narrative demonstrates how the fields of science, engineering, law, and medicine interconnect. *Vanishing Bone* will inspire with its proof of the ways that scientific research impacts lives."

—KIMBERLY WRIGHT CASSIDY, *President and Professor of Psychology, Bryn Mawr College*

"*Vanishing Bone* is a story that illustrates the power of careful clinical observation, rigorous interdisciplinary science, innovation, and research translation to improve human health. This book is a testament to the impactful role the author has had on the field of joint replacement surgery and his tireless dedication to his patients. This volume will be of interest not only to joint replacement surgeons, but also to the larger medical community and any individual interested in a good medical mystery."

—JOSHUA JACOBS, MD, *William A. Hark, MD/Susanne G. Swift Professor and Chairman, Department of Orthopaedic Surgery, Rush University Medical Center*

VANISHING BONE

Conquering a Stealth Disease
Caused by Total Hip Replacements

William H. Harris, MD, DSc

OXFORD
UNIVERSITY PRESS

OXFORD
UNIVERSITY PRESS

Oxford University Press is a department of the University of Oxford. It furthers the University's objective of excellence in research, scholarship, and education by publishing worldwide. Oxford is a registered trade mark of Oxford University Press in the UK and certain other countries.

Published in the United States of America by Oxford University Press 198 Madison Avenue, New York, NY 10016, United States of America.

© Oxford University Press 2018

All rights reserved. No part of this publication may be reproduced, stored in a retrieval system, or transmitted, in any form or by any means, without the prior permission in writing of Oxford University Press, or as expressly permitted by law, by license, or under terms agreed with the appropriate reproduction rights organization. Inquiries concerning reproduction outside the scope of the above should be sent to the Rights Department, Oxford University Press, at the address above.

You must not circulate this work in any other form and you must impose this same condition on any acquirer.

Library of Congress Cataloging-in-Publication Data
Names: Harris, William H. (William Hamilton), 1927– author.
Title: Vanishing bone : conquering a stealth disease caused by total hip replacements / William H. Harris, MD, DSc.
Description: New York, NY : Oxford University Press, [2018]
Identifiers: LCCN 2017004759 | ISBN 9780190687762 (hardback)
Subjects: LCSH: Total hip replacement. | Bone resorption.
Classification: LCC RD549 .H38 2017 | DDC 617.5/810592—dc23
LC record available at https://lccn.loc.gov/2017004759

This material is not intended to be, and should not be considered, a substitute for medical or other professional advice. Treatment for the conditions described in this material is highly dependent on the individual circumstances. And, while this material is designed to offer accurate information with respect to the subject matter covered and to be current as of the time it was written, research and knowledge about medical and health issues is constantly evolving and dose schedules for medications are being revised continually, with new side effects recognized and accounted for regularly. Readers must therefore always check the product information and clinical procedures with the most up-to-date published product information and data sheets provided by the manufacturers and the most recent codes of conduct and safety regulation. The publisher and the authors make no representations or warranties to readers, express or implied, as to the accuracy or completeness of this material. Without limiting the foregoing, the publisher and the authors make no representations or warranties as to the accuracy or efficacy of the drug dosages mentioned in the material. The authors and the publisher do not accept, and expressly disclaim, any responsibility for any liability, loss or risk that may be claimed or incurred as a consequence of the use and/or application of any of the contents of this material.

1 3 5 7 9 8 6 4 2
Printed by Sheridan Books, Inc., United States of America

To Nan

A most beautiful person, on the outside and deep inside.

CONTENTS

PART TWO Final Hurdles

FOREWORD

BY EDWARD O. WILSON

An understanding of science, sorely needed throughout the world, cannot be achieved merely by learning the facts and theories produced by scientists. It demands, as well, a clear image of the process of scientific research, which in turn calls for knowledge of the way in which scientific thinking resembles other more ordinary processes of the human mind, and ways in which it differs.

True scientific research can be viewed as an adventure of another kind. There exists a mystery to be solved, a problem of a kind that matters, an opportunity, a rare chance to enter wholly new territory, the thrill of being the first to see something completely new. We all love adventures, and in science, we enjoy them most if told by the scientists who lived them.

So how can you tell whether the writer is authentic? A true scientist, as opposed to a journalist, historian, or popular writer, however gifted, is one who can finish the following sentence relative to the story: "I discovered that (or I led the team that) . . . ." If the tale unfolds thus, and is on a subject of importance to a great many people, the denouement may not be just riveting, but historic in its own right.

These rare qualities come together in William H. Harris' *Vanishing Bone*. He led the team that contributed much to the diagnosis—and then provided a cure—of the bone-dissolving disease periprosthetic osteolysis (bone destruction) that crippled thousands and threatened millions more. To achieve success, Harris and his coworkers engaged in the kinds of thought processes and endeavors it takes to make a major scientific advance.

The subject, although on a thoroughly medical topic that at first might seem arcane, in fact is a mystery of the first rank. Readers will not be on a search for pirate gold or the headwaters of a lost river, but this story is fundamentally the same. Clues or leads are followed, hopes are raised and sometimes dashed, until, finally, the great is achieved.

Vanishing Bone is an equally good read under a beach umbrella or for a university seminar.

This is the story of the virtually complete eradication of a disease never seen before in the long history of humankind. Ironically, it was created, inadvertently, by surgeons. From its first appearance in 1958 until its elimination in 2000, the disease was disastrous for many thousands of people and seriously disrupted the lives of more than a million. The disease destroyed the bone around total hip and total knee replacements.

Its jaw-breaking name, *periprosthetic* (around the prosthesis) *osteolysis* (bone destruction), was not then, is not now, and never will become a household phrase. Yet, in its extreme form, for one patient, for example, it required replacement of a large segment of the pelvis and the upper half of the femur with bony parts borrowed from a bone bank.

In the beginning, doctors thought this severe erosion of bone was a rare anomaly, but soon this insidious disease would be the number-one reason for failure of hip replacements around the world. Orthopaedic surgeons everywhere were desperate to find a cure.

To defeat this dire disease, we first had to solve the mystery of what it was. For that, we needed the dogged determination of a detective—at the cellular and molecular levels. After we identified the culprit causing the destruction, we turned our skills to invention, using the latest techniques of polymer science to create an entirely new material to thwart the destruction.

From the time of our initial observation of this disease, we faced one unanticipated hurdle after another. We were forced to go beyond the limits of known medical science to stop this devastating disease, and the stakes were high. With hundreds of thousands of people each year in need of hip replacements, and an increasing overall number of patients at risk, failure was not an option. Our success meant restoring the majesty of this "spectacular but dangerous" operation called *total hip replacement*.

One further preamble. Readers should not anticipate that *Vanishing Bone* represents an unbiased, historical account of the totality of the scientific effort to unravel this bone-destroying disease and the invention of crosslinked polyethylene for medical use. Rather, it is predominantly the reflection of the tortuous experience of our laboratory in our trek to uncover and overcome an unknown, unique disease.

For example, after the identification by my research team of two compounds produced by the cellular activity of the key cells in this disease—the macrophages—the pursuit of the detailed molecular biology causing the disease engaged many laboratories around the world, including, among many others, the research group at Rush Medical School in Chicago, Illinois (Tibor T. Glant, Arum Shanbhag, J. J. Jacobs, J. Galante, and others); the University of California, Los Angeles, California (Harlan Amstutz and others); Rochester Medical School, Rochester, New York (E. M. Schwarz, R. W. Rosier, and R. J. O'Keefe); the research group at Washington University, St. Louis, Missouri (with J. C. Clohisy and S. L. Teitelbaum); Stanford University, Stanford, California (S. B. Goodman);

University of Pittsburgh, Pittsburgh, Pennsylvania (Harry Rubash); and many others. Because the exquisite explanation of the molecular biology revealed much about the mechanism of the disease, but did *not* lead to a discrete treatment or prevention of the disease, I did not include the fine details of that outstanding science in this book. Instead, I concentrated on issues related directly to the elimination of periprosthetic osteolysis.

The names and identifying details of the patients mentioned in this book have been changed, but the facts and conclusions are all based on real cases. Dialogues recreated for the purposes of narration also approximate what actually happened to the best of my memory.

A second disclaimer is this. The first 18 years of experience using crosslinked polyethylene have been virtually free of cases of bone destruction. This is a very strong record, reflecting its use by an estimated seven million patients. Nevertheless, until even more years pass, we will not know with absolute certainty that late cases of bone destruction or even some other unanticipated adverse effect might arise.

Because this adventure covers four decades, a "timeline" is provided on pages xxi–xxii.

Here is my story.

LIST OF FIGURES AND TABLES

Figures

Tables

AN EXPLANATION OF KEY TERMS

Naturally, a few terms or concepts may be unfamiliar to you at first. Fear not. This problem is easily overcome.

This mysterious disease produced very extensive destruction of bone next to the artificial parts of total hip replacements. The only cells in the body with the capacity to destroy bone are called *osteoclasts*. (*Osteo* refers to "bone" and *clast* means "eat away.") The other cell involved in this disease, which is the primary culprit behind the disease, has the curious name *macrophage*. *Macro* means "big," and *phage* means "eater." And these cells are truly *big eaters*. They are one type of the body's defense cells and they eat things such as bacteria. These are the only two cells you meet in this book.

I also talk about a plastic called *polyethylene*. You probably already know some polyethylenes because of their widespread use in daily life. The form of polyethylene to which I refer is somewhat different, because it is made of very, very long and very, very thin strands that are arranged somewhat like a pile of spaghetti in a bowl.

As we begin to unravel the scientific mystery of this disease and find a cure, I describe a process of bonding, or *linking,* one strand of the polyethylene to the adjacent strand. Because these bonds occur across many strands of polyethylene, the whole process is known as *crosslinking.* As you will see, *crosslinked polyethylene* is the key to the cure of the disease.

TIMELINE OF KEY EVENTS

1957	John Charnley introduced total hip replacement (THR) using Teflon-like plastic in nearly 300 cases.
1958–1960	Nearly 300 failed, badly.
1962	John Charnley reintroduced THR using polyethylene.
1974	I saw my first four cases of massive bone destruction around THR. The biopsies showed "sheets of macrophages and massive bone destruction." Published in 1976.
1974	Willert proposed the critical explanation of what was happening, suggesting the macrophages were attracted to eliminate tiny particles of the bone cement used to fix the THR components to the bone.
1980–1984	Cementless total hips were introduced to circumvent the need for bone cement.
1987	Publication of an article titled "Cement Disease."
1990	Our discovery of bone destruction among cementless THR. This observation forced the "cement disease" concept to be enlarged to include particles of polyethylene, and the disease to be renamed "particle disease."
1990	Bone destruction became fully recognized as the dominant, long-term cause of failure of THR worldwide.
1990	We initiated our quest for a better articulation for THR, but started with the unexpected search for a more sophisticated hip simulator.

1993	Our original observation was made showing the reorientation of the polyethylene molecules because of gait, leading to our hypothesis that crosslinking might prevent wear.
1995	Ed Merrill of the Massachusetts Institute of Technology "recommended crosslinking the polyethylene using electron beam irradiation to prevent the reorientation of the strands of polyethylene."
1995	Early attempts at crosslinking the polyethylene produced melting, fires, and explosions.
1995	Effective crosslinking was achieved without melting, fires, or explosions.
1995	Presentation to the US Food and Drug Administration was interrupted by a bomb threat.
1995	Licensed with Sulzer, Inc.
1995	Negotiated with Johnson & Johnson.
1995	Licensed with Zimmer, Inc.
1998, December	The first human implantation of highly crosslinked polyethylene was performed.
1998, December	Radiostereometric analysis studies of our crosslinked polyethylene began in Goteborg, Sweden.
2002	Sulzer goes bankrupt.
2003	Zimmer buys Sulzer (Centerpulse).
1999–2016	An estimated six million patients get highly crosslinked THR.
2017	Bone destruction around total hip replacements has been eliminated.

VANISHING BONE

PART I

Astonishing Discoveries

To raise new questions, new possibilities, to regard old problems from a new angle, requires creative imagination and marks real advances in science.

—ALBERT EINSTEIN

Chapter 1

The Game Is Afoot!

I didn't think. I investigated.

—WILHELM RÖNTGEN, *Nobel laureate,*
when asked what he thought when
he first discovered the x-ray

For 40 years I investigated a baffling medical mystery—one that would reveal a totally new disease never seen before in the history of humankind.

It all started with a single x-ray.

When I first saw him in November 1974, Peter Dunn, 55, was a West Coast attorney accustomed to striding across courtrooms and winning multimillion-dollar lawsuits. His extraordinary confidence and well-tailored suits gave him an unmistakable aura of success, but by the time he arrived in my office, he couldn't stride across the room to shake my hand. He limped.

"About eight years ago I was taking a long deposition in San Diego," Peter told me. "When we broke for lunch, my hip was so stiff I could barely stand up! Before long, I started having trouble climbing stairs. It only got worse from there," he shrugged, cutting to the chase. "Eventually, my doctor recommended total hip replacement surgery."

"Which you had seven years ago?" I confirmed, looking at his records.

"Yes. It was a great relief at first; but lately, when I walk, my hip feels—I don't know how to say this—kind of *loose*. It hurts to put weight on it. The pain is so bad I can barely sleep at night. Sometimes it radiates halfway down my leg." He winced as he rubbed his left thigh.

"No one I've consulted has been able to help. I'm hoping you can. The orthopaedic surgeons in San Francisco told me you have a reputation for fixing hip replacements that go wrong. They said you find solutions others can't. You're a research scientist."

"A clinician–scientist," I explained. "I have a very active clinical practice as the chief of hip surgery at the Massachusetts General Hospital (MGH), but I also run an extensive research lab, which I founded for the purpose of finding solutions to problems with hip replacements that haven't been solved before."

"First, I'd like to do a physical exam," I told him, "then we'll get an x-ray."

When radiology sent the x-ray to me, I was shocked. I wasn't even sure what I was looking at. In thousands of x-rays of patients with hip replacements, I'd never seen anything like it before. My heart raced and my mind blurted, "Oh my God. This must be cancer." The image of the thigh piece of the hip prosthesis appeared in the x-ray in stark white, as it should, but alongside it were dozens of gaping black areas—holes in the femur. Some kind of a very rapid, aggressive process was destroying vast amounts of Peter's bone. Whole chunks of the femur were completely gone. What on Earth could be causing this? (See Figure 1.1.)

Ordinarily, when a bone is destroyed from an injury or an infection, new bone begins to reform very quickly. The same thing happens with many cancers; the body responds to the attack. But Peter's body was not fighting back. It seemed to be making no attempt to repair itself at all.

The logical deduction was cancer, but it didn't fit. Cancer almost never occurs around a total hip prosthesis. It just doesn't happen. For a long time, hip surgeons worried about that risk because we were putting into the body a huge, foreign device that would release low levels of ions for years to come. It was only natural to be concerned about cancer. As a result, the fate of total hip replacement's relation to the occurrence of cancer had been closely monitored since the inception of total hip surgery. There had never been any correlation between cancer and a hip replacement—unless that's what I was looking at in Peter's x-ray. Still, it didn't make sense.

Bone cancer is certainly capable of this magnitude of aggressive bone destruction, but primary bone cancer is extremely rare and it doesn't occur around the hip in middle-aged men. The likelihood that Peter had developed two rare conditions—cancer

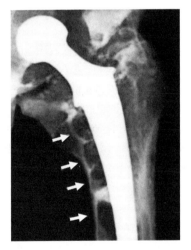

FIGURE 1.1 *Dark Areas of Bone Destruction*

X-ray of the left hip seven years after a total hip replacement, showing the metal thigh piece as the long white object in the center of the thigh bone, or femur. The dark areas in the bone (arrows) are regions where bone had previously been, but all of that bone was completely destroyed.

around a prosthesis *and* bone cancer at this location at middle age—was virtually nil.

Mystified, I reviewed all of Peter's medical history and previous x-rays again, hoping to find clues, but found none. It was frustrating to have so little information. As unlikely as it seemed, cancer was still the best candidate by a huge margin. Secondary cancers are those that start somewhere else in the body and spread to the femur. Despite my doubts, my working hypothesis was that this had to be a type of secondary cancer. It was the only thing I'd ever seen that could destroy that much bone with no reaction.

"I'm very sorry to give you news that might have serious consequences," I told Peter. "The x-ray is inconclusive. We'll need to do a full battery of tests."

Peter was rightfully concerned, and he braced himself for bad news, but the test results revealed no evidence of cancer or any other disease—anywhere in his body!

I took the case to Grand Rounds.

Since Grand Rounds began at Johns Hopkins in 1889, they have been a tradition at every academic medical center. Physicians present cases to the medical staff, residents, interns, and medical students in their specialty. Each case is laid out with its perplexities, successes, or failures and then possible diagnoses are avidly discussed by everyone from the most distinguished surgeons to the newest recruits. Arguments and disagreements sometimes result in a lively debate, but the ability to tap into that collective font of knowledge is priceless.

Most of medicine occurs in one-on-one exchanges between patients and doctors in the privacy of a medical office. In contrast, Grand Rounds offer the invaluable opportunity of garnering the accumulated wisdom of 100 colleagues or so with the same passionate commitment to orthopaedics. It's an extraordinarily powerful resource for education and the refined development of thought. Enormous learning takes place. In my view, it reaches its greatest majesty on unusual cases. Any experienced doctor can give feedback about ordinary cases, but it's the problems that few people have ever encountered before that yield the greatest benefits from Grand Rounds. Among the most experienced surgeons, even their guesses are well-informed.

From the time I was a beginning resident in 1955 watching the senior staff of the Orthopaedic Department of the MGH present the cases that stumped them, there were always three or four of the more experienced senior staff members who would say, "Oh, yes! I had a case like this 20 years ago. It turned out to be X." Or "I was once involved in a research project where two out of 40 subjects had this type of condition and these were the results." Whatever it was, someone would have seen it. And these people were talkers. Like all surgeons accustomed to making life-and-death decisions every day, they held strong opinions they were not reluctant to express.

So it came as a surprise when, after I'd detailed Peter's case and placed the last x-ray on the viewbox on the stage of the Bigelow Amphitheater, I was met with silence. No one on the entire staff had ever seen anything like this x-ray before. Bone destruction, yes. But not alongside a prosthesis. Wear and tear, of course. But not an alarming cluster of holes in the bone that had made the thigh piece of the total hip replacement loose and threatened to undermine the integrity of the femur with no evidence of cancer anywhere in the body.

When they did start talking, they scrambled through the same thoughts I'd had: "But there's no evidence of cancer being caused by prostheses!" "How could it be bone cancer anyway in a middle-aged man at this location?" And, most confusing of all,

"Why wasn't the bone fighting back?" We discussed the possibilities for the remainder of the hour. The final consensus was to stop the speculation, get a piece of tissue, and find out exactly what was going on.

What in the world was this?

Chapter 2

The Cart Before the Horse

*The cart has been put before the horse. The artificial joint has been
made and used. Now we are trying to find out how and why it fails.*
— SIR JOHN CHARNLEY, *Founder of total hip replacement surgery*

The biopsy results were stunning. No cancer cells of any type.
Not even a benign tumor. No infection at all. Even worse, Peter
Dunn's biopsy showed no other recognizable disease! This
was something none of us had ever seen before: the aggressive
destruction of bone near the prosthesis—in a totally healthy
adult male.

Even the terms the pathologist used to describe the biopsy
were strange. He said the tissue alongside the "aggressive bone
destruction" consisted of "sheets of macrophages." Macrophages
are a type of white blood cell and are the body's scavenger cells;
they attack and digest bacteria, foreign substances, and dead and
dying cells. Normally existing in small numbers in almost every
tissue, they can also travel throughout the body to accumulate
wherever needed, and they are also crucial to initiating certain
aspects of the body's immune response.

It would not be surprising to find macrophages swarming to
the site of an infection, but the blood tests and fluid from the
hip joint confirmed there was no infection in Peter's hip. Why
were they there at all, much less in such huge numbers? Virtually
all the cells in the entire biopsy were macrophages. This was

unprecedented. There was no known disease for which all the tissue consisted of macrophages. Incidentally, the translation of the term *macrophage* is "big eater," because the way they attack bacteria or dead cells is actually by ingesting them. That is to say, these cells can physically take the bacteria or dead cells into the interior of the macrophage itself and eradicate them inside their cell wall (Figures 2.1 and 2.2).

Whatever was going on, the macrophages had not simply rushed to the area to fend off an infection or clean up dead cells. For some reason, they had banded together to form a solid sheet of rubbery tissue that lay adjacent to the bone, and the bone itself was being aggressively resorbed or "eaten away," according to the pathologist.

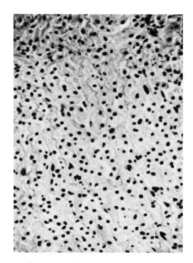

FIGURE 2.1 *Sheets of Macrophages*

Photomicrograph (a photo through a microscope) showing only one type of cell: the *macrophage*. This appearance was described by the pathologist as "sheets of macrophages."

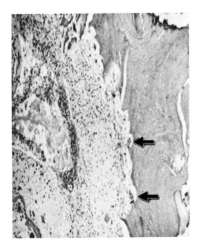

FIGURE 2.2 *Bone Destruction*

Photomicrograph showing gray material at the right edge (bone) with bone-eating cells (osteoclasts) aggressively eating the bone (arrows).

But only one type of cell in the body can resorb bone: a different cell called an *osteoclast*.

Normally, osteoclasts nibble at the bone, taking microscopic bites along the edge of the cell. Like a mouse eating a big chunk of cheese, you know they've been there because they leave a hollowed out divot in the bone. No other cell can take away bone.

But these osteoclasts weren't just nibbling at Peter's thigh bone, they were gutting it, wrapped in inexplicable sheets of macrophages no one had ever seen before. It was as if the normal process of bone resorption had gone wild. We had no previous information to work with. We couldn't build a hypothesis based on similar cases, because there were none. Until this biopsy, we had never seen masses of macrophages associated with huge bone resorption in any way. To call it bizarre was an understatement.

Since my earliest days in medical training, it has always been my habit to go to the pathology lab and get the pathologist to show me firsthand what he was looking at and to hear what he was thinking. This process has enhanced my comprehension enormously. I learned it at my dad's knee. In his medical practice, even though he was a radiologist, he followed the basic ancient dictum: Go see the patient. If he was uncertain about what an x-ray showed, he'd always go see the patient. He taught me, "If you're trying to solve a mystery, you've got to see it for yourself."

But in this case, even that didn't help. I didn't even know how to start thinking about it. First, we had those startling x-rays, then the pathology results. Pathology reports usually tell you what's going on, but this time they only deepened the mystery. Now we had this nutty combination of cells with no relationship to anything we knew about.

Initially, I drew a blank; then I got speculative. That was exciting. During the previous 12 years, starting in 1962, many thousands of similar total hip replacements had been done worldwide. So, this must have been seen before. In all that time, I thought, surely other surgeons must have come across a similar reaction. But I couldn't help but wonder if the first one to see it was the very surgeon who invented hip replacements: Sir John Charnley (Profile 2.1).

It is widely believed that John Charnley invented total hip replacement when, in 1962, he performed the first total hip replacement surgery using a polyethylene plastic to replace the cartilage in the hip. But in fact, the operation in 1962 was, in reality, a *reintroduction* of the concept; the first of this type of operation had been done by Charnley five years earlier, in 1957. However, at that time, the cartilage was replaced by a different plastic called *PTFE*, which we know as Teflon. That difference is important because of the fate of that plastic.

PROFILE 2.1   Sir John Charnley

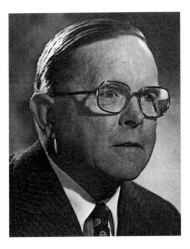

Reprinted with permission from Debbie McGowan, editor, Beaten Track Publishing, Burscough, Lancashire, UK.

Sir John Charnley (1918–1982) was the most innovative orthopaedic surgeon of all time.

That's a very strong statement, but it's backed by facts. His creative, persistent, resilient, and insightful activities were dominant contributions to the entire field of orthopaedic surgery. Almost single-handedly, he generated the entire realm of extraordinarily effective therapeutics known as *total joint surgery*. It is hard to imagine total hip surgery, total knee surgery, total elbow surgery, and the rest of total joint surgery without his contributions.

Were that not enough, he made major world-class contributions to tribology (the study of the function of joints); his book on the management of fractures, *The Closed Treatment of Common Fractures*, is outstanding; he created very impressive work on the fusion of joints; and his contributions to the prevention of infections in surgical wounds were remarkable. His laser-like focus and monolithic dedication are inspirational.

Few surgeons could respond as he did to his first experience of the nearly 300 consecutive *failures* of his heavily criticized, totally unsupported radical new idea in hip surgery. After being forced to reoperate on nearly all of his first 300 *unsuccessful* patients who received his original Teflon-like total hip replacement, he responded with renewed dedication, reinforced by the belief that—at the heart of these failures—he envisioned a majestic solution.

From the point of view of *creativity*, he demonstrated a uniquely effective combination of having an inspired visionary concept that he blended intimately with the rigorous quantification of every element involved in his subsequent successes and failures.

His 1979 book *Low Friction Arthroplasty of the Hip* is a classic. The world owes him a huge measure of gratitude.

He received the Lasker Award in 1974, commonly called the American Nobel Prize, and was knighted by Queen Elizabeth in 1977. He was elected to membership in the Royal Society.

The striking initial success of Charnley's revolutionary operation with the PTFE total hip was extraordinary; some said miraculous. It was the first time anyone had ever replaced the whole hip joint in the human body with metal and plastic materials. Skeptics countered that these plastic joints wouldn't last, but his patients were elated by the results. After suffering desperately from severe pain and poor mobility for years, they were finally pain free and able to walk, even dance.

Sadly, those initial successes were short-lived. Within a year or two, the PTFE had worn badly. Every single one of the first nearly 300 total hip replacements using PTFE failed—and failed badly, causing severe pain and an ugly limp. The entire artificial joint had to be taken out with nothing to put back in its place.

The failure was devastating for the nearly 300 patients who were left with no hip joint whatsoever—and for Charnley. Redoubling his efforts, Charnley began laboratory experiments with many other plastics, culminating in the selection of a more durable plastic: a polyethylene. By November 1962, his experiments convinced him that this polyethylene would, in fact, work.

It was in 1965, during the early period of polyethylene total hips, that I first met Charnley while I was on a prestigious American–British–Canadian Traveling Fellowship. Four of us from the United States, all of whom were younger than 40 years old and yet considered to be the next leaders in orthopaedics, had been selected by the American Orthopaedic Association for this fellowship to travel throughout Great Britain to study British orthopaedic techniques. We visited Charnley at the partially abandoned hospital he had resurrected in Lancashire, United Kingdom. We had the privilege of watching him operate. It was the first time I'd seen a total hip replacement and I was astonished.

The relief of pain and the superb quality of life that were the results of total hip replacement were completely unprecedented.

In the years to come, he and I appeared together in many orthopaedic programs at meetings around the world, and I got to know him well. If anyone had observed this extraordinary bone destruction that we were seeing in Peter Dunn's case, it would be Charnley.

I combed through his publications again, looking for any mention of bone destruction or macrophages near the site of a total hip replacement. And then I found it. In some of his later reports of the 300 PTFE hip replacement surgeries that failed, Charnley noted a few instances in which the pelvis, the femur, or both showed the same kind of bone destruction we were seeing in Peter!

Only a handful of people in the world had seen this phenomenon, but the man who had been doing hip replacements the longest was among them and had been the first. Finally, I had confirmation. I was not the only person to see this bizarre and alarming situation.

But unfortunately, Charnley's experiences didn't help resolve our dilemma, and for three very different reasons. The first was Charnley's wise decision not to allow anyone else to do his radical new PTFE surgery until he had confirmed its reliability. Because it did not prove to be reliable, he was the only surgeon in the world who had personally witnessed bone destruction at that time. Therefore, no one else had seen the bone destruction from PTFE.

His successful search for a better material led to a polyethylene, the remarkable effectiveness of which was the second reason we were ignorant of details about such bone destruction. No patient who got the polyethylene implant showed any bone destruction, even after five or six years. The early operations using polyethylene replacements were a heartening success. And even those surgeons who, by the late 1960s, had heard of the bone destruction around the PTFE total hips were fully reassured, because it did not occur with the polyethylene cases. So, the success of the polyethylene total hips diverted concerns about the fact that some of the PTFE patients had shown bone destruction.

The third reason that concern about the bone destruction issue was dormant was perhaps the strangest. Charnley, erroneously, felt these unusual cases of bone destruction in the PTFE cases were caused by infection. This was because, at the initiation of this unique type of surgery, which introduced into the body such a huge foreign implant, Charnley's infection rate was nearly 10%. That was a very serious and remarkably high rate. Because infection can cause major bone destruction, Charnley attributed all these cases of bone destruction around the PTFE total hip replacements to infection.

Curiously, he came to this conclusion despite the fact that his tests for bacteria in the wound were negative. He was not even able to grow any bacteria in any of his tests of the surrounding tissue, nor could he see any evidence of infection under the microscope. As I now knew from Peter Dunn's case, what he was looking at was inexplicable, but his best guess was that these were cases of occult infection.

As was also typical of this great innovator, Charnley acted on his conviction that invisible bacteria were contaminating hip surgery. Imaginatively, he developed (1) an air filtration system to isolate the wound in the operating theater and (2) a ventilated operating gown to prevent bacterial contamination from the surgeons. Both are still in use today.

The massive bone destruction accompanying hip replacements in a *polyethylene* total hip, with which I was now confronted, was a different and disturbing story (see Figures 2.3–2.5). Uncertainty

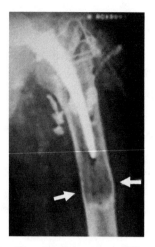

FIGURE 2.3 *Extensive Bone Destruction of Femur*

This x-ray shows extensive destruction in the femur, around the femoral component and below (arrows).

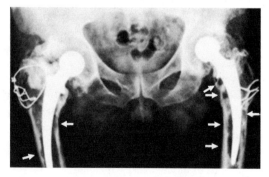

FIGURE 2.4 *Bone Destruction in Both Femurs*

This x-ray shows extensive bone destruction in each femur around the femoral prosthesis (arrows). Reprinted with permission from Wolters Kluwer Health, Inc. from *Journal of Bone and Joint Surgery* 58-A(5), fig 2, page 614, July 1976.

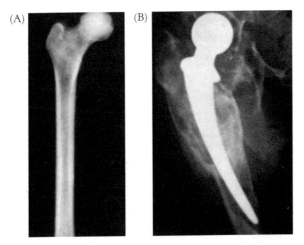

FIGURE 2.5 *Normal Femur and Femur Distorted by Bone Destruction*

This pair of x-rays shows the destructive power of this disease. Contrast the normal femur (A) with the massively distorted femur that resulted from the effects of the bone destruction and subsequent bone remodeling over time (B).

prevailed. No one had a clue what this bone destruction was or how to prevent it. Over time, other surgeons offered theories to explain this rare but alarming phenomenon. A few suggested that mechanical factors, such as the chronic rubbing of a loose component against the bone, might be to blame. An adverse reaction, such as an allergy to bone cement, was also considered.

I was determined that I had to uncover the source of the problem and resolve it, or at least take a crack at it. The stakes were just too high to do anything less.

Not long after Peter Dunn's mysterious case appeared, three very similar cases crossed my desk. Two were my own patients for whom I had done total hip replacements. As an aside, these two cases increased the impact on me of these previously unheard-of scenarios. Although I felt full and keen responsibility to exert maximum effort to try to solve Peter's problem, these two additional cases raised my emotional link and responsibility commitment even higher just because I was the surgeon responsible for doing their original total hip operations. All four cases showed the same "aggressive bone destruction with sheets of macrophages."

Hoping to alert the field of hip surgery to my findings and focus worldwide attention on this disturbing problem, my article about these four cases was published in the *Journal of Bone and Joint Surgery,* the recognized leader among the orthopaedic scientific journals of the day, in 1976. There was little response to this article, because most hip surgeons around the world were completely unaware of this condition. I was beginning to think the condition had to be an mysterious but unique *disease,* rather than just a sporadic or isolated manifestation of, for example, a local toxic reaction to the mere presence of the implants.

The *Journal* published the article perhaps somewhat as an oddity. The publication of these four strange cases was a measure of the widespread ignorance about this condition at the time. It stands in sharp contrast to the fact that, in the decades since, surgeons would come to identify this bone destruction around prostheses of total hip replacements and total knee replacements in tens of thousands of patients—*well in excess of a million patients!*

Chapter 3

Uniquely Creative, But Dangerous

The science of today is the technology of tomorrow.
—EDWARD TELLER

Total hip replacement is one of the most dramatic revolutions in the long history of human surgery. It has revitalized lives, eliminated pain, and restored mobility to so many millions of people that, today, the marvel of this surgery has become almost commonplace. But, to consider it ordinary is to miss the sheer wonder of this procedure.

There is no denying the fact that an invasion of the body of this magnitude in the treatment of arthritis is extreme. It requires the entire removal of the upper end of the thigh bone. Sharp power tools are used aggressively to reshape the entire hip socket. A huge and complex metal and plastic hip joint is then installed into the bones and nestled into the living tissues of the human body. It literally gives patients the kind of bionic enhancements that are often the subject of science fiction.

While I was delighted to see this transformation in my patients, it was especially gratifying when I was able to bring this marvelous enhancement to a dear friend. At my local tennis club, I was often paired, during in the early '70s, with Karl Edelman in Men's Doubles for the round-robin events on Sunday mornings. Our tennis skills were well-matched, which made for great teamwork when we played together—and a stimulating challenge when we played against each other.

In 1939, Karl had immigrated to the United States. With his gregarious personality, he easily built a successful series of real estate brokerage firms along the East Coast.

The first sign of trouble came when Karl's tennis game hit a slump. He'd always had a great backhand, but more and more he caught the ball too late, and a bit later on he began to miss it altogether! Shots he'd normally return with gusto flew past him on the court unchallenged. To compensate, he stopped playing singles while he worked on his speed and agility, but pain soon stopped him altogether.

His wife, Ingrid, started to notice that it was becoming common to find Karl frowning and massaging his hip. One day, when he came off the court to meet her for lunch, he startled her. "Are you *limping?*" she asked.

That's when he came to see me. Although he had done a remarkable job of pushing through it, Karl was experiencing severe bilateral hip pain that not only impaired his daily activities, but also affected the management of his businesses as well. I spoke to his wife and him about what a total hip replacement could do to alleviate his pain.

Ingrid reacted with alarm. She was quite concerned about the surgery. My assurances helped soothe her, but it was the encouragement of their friends with hip implants at the tennis club that had the most impact. Many of them had had similar apprehensions, but had come to realize their fears were unwarranted. Although major surgery was indeed stressful, it bore no comparison to the nightmares of a vivid imagination.

Karl was less anxious about the operation than Ingrid, but as a precaution, we decided to do one hip first and then wait until he was ready to proceed with the other.

After seeing the delight and enthusiasm of thousands of patients after this surgery, I could have predicted what would happen next. Both Karl and Ingrid were startled by his new mobility and lack of pain. The contrast of the stiff, untreated, arthritic hip to the perfectly functioning, painless hip was suddenly cast in sharp relief. Karl couldn't wait to do the other hip! By the time he had recovered from that second operation, Karl was a new man. His only regret was that he hadn't done the operation sooner! No one was more surprised and delighted than Ingrid.

My real joy came in watching Karl on the courts from the viewing gallery after we completed that second surgery. Not only did he move like a spry, much younger man, but he'd started playing singles again—and was winning!

Although, of course, it's something of an overstatement, it was experiences like these that made me tell a friend on one of those special, really good days in my office, "I see only two kinds of people: patients who are waiting for a total hip replacement and patients who are happy!"

After the astonishing installation of such a huge foreign joint, many patients have a very striking and complete relief of pain. In today's world (although not so during the early days of total hip replacement), younger patients are frequently rapidly back on the golf course or able to play tennis. This level of function and freedom from pain were completely inconceivable before the introduction of total hip replacement surgery. To appreciate the full magnitude of this momentous invention, it is important also to acknowledge the extraordinary parallel advances that total hip replacement has spawned in the treatment of severe arthritis of knees, ankles, shoulders, and elbows.

All this is in sharp contrast to hip surgery before total hip replacement. Then, only three operations existed for patients with advanced arthritis of the hip: hip fusion (making the hip completely stiff), osteotomy of the hip (dividing the femur not far below the ball to allow the ball to spin enough to bring undamaged cartilage into the joint), and cup arthroplasty (removing the damaged cartilage and encouraging new cartilage to grow). All three of these operations had marked limitations. Osteotomies eventually wore out. Many cup arthroplasty operations resulted in a failure to grow sufficient new cartilage to afford patients a pain-free and functional hip. All three operations required long hospitalizations with extended rehabilitation periods. Moreover, neither osteotomy nor hip fusion were suitable for patients with rheumatoid arthritis of the hip.

But, with total hip replacement, the arthritis is completely cut out and replaced with a brand new artificial hip joint. For the patient, there is an exhilarating relief from pain and a marvelous restoration of motion and function. In short, total hip replacement is a uniquely creative and highly rewarding operation. But it is simultaneously highly dangerous.

Highly rewarding? Yes. Highly dangerous? Yes, indeed. When successful total hip surgery was first introduced during the 1960s, even we surgeons who were recommending this surgery did not, at that time, fully appreciate how dangerous it was.

To excise the entire hip joint and replace it with massive metal and plastic parts was audacious, and quite risky. For example, the infection rate—an infected total hip operation is a terrible problem—was frighteningly high: initially about 10%. Some of the metal thigh pieces broke. Many, many of the thigh pieces and socket pieces came loose from the bone and were painful, and yet another operation was required. The artificial hip could dislocate; that is to say, the ball slipped out of the joint, catapulting the unsuspecting patient to the floor. And death? Yes, death occurred, most commonly from a pulmonary embolus.

I learned , in concept, about the risk of dying from a pulmonary embolus while I was in medical school, but my *real* education about how devastating a fatal pulmonary embolism could be occurred when I was chief orthopaedic resident at the MGH in 1959. I was totally unprepared for the profound effect of this complication.

Blood clots can form in the veins of the calf or thigh under many different circumstances, most often in patients who are older, who have cancer, or who have hip surgery. A blood clot that passes from the leg of the patient into the lungs, called a *pulmonary embolus*, can block the blood supply to the lungs. If the blockage is great enough, the patient will not survive.

In 1959, because successful total hip replacement surgery had yet to be invented, I performed a cup arthroplasty on the right hip of my patient, Tom Martin. For the management of his equally severe arthritis in the opposite hip, I performed a similar operation on his left hip two weeks later. During that surgery, his blood pressure suddenly dropped to zero.

This was a total surprise. We had no explanation. The anesthesia had appeared to be quite satisfactory up to that point. Bleeding at the wound had been minimal. He had no known heart disease.

I took immediate action, rapidly closing the wound and using every method I knew to restore his blood pressure. Despite these efforts, he died in my arms.

Although I knew full well that all major surgery carried with it severe risks, I was decimated. With utter dismay, I informed his wife and his two young children in the waiting room that, instead of helping, my surgery had taken the life of their loved one. And it ruined their own lives. I struggled mightily to compose myself after this horrifying loss.

This tragedy was compounded by the fact that Tom was such a loving husband and father—a perfectly wonderful man. Even with a modest education he had created a stable family as a day laborer, buying a portion of a three-decker home, and becoming a responsible citizen in his community. He dreamed that eventually he would be able to send his children to college so they would have opportunities he never had. With his sudden, unforeseen death, all these plans were snuffed out.

The postmortem examination showed Thomas had had a massive pulmonary embolism from a clot in his calf that started after the first operation. At that singular moment, I quietly resolved to do whatever I could to prevent such a catastrophe from ever occurring again.

Despite my determination, I had to admit that the possibility of me fulfilling my vow seemed unlikely. I was a young, widely unknown, orthopaedic surgeon who had not even completed his training. Moreover, pulmonary embolisms were the purview of hematologists and lung physicians, not orthopaedic surgeons. At that time, during the late 1950s, even *those* specialists had no way to diagnose a blood clot in a calf, and no way to prevent fatal pulmonary emboli.

Thus, I was particularly appalled by the very high rate of fatal pulmonary emboli following total hip replacement surgery during the early 1960s. One patient out of every 50 patients after a total hip replacement died of a fatal pulmonary embolus! This was a huge risk. And this risk was taken in the treatment of arthritis, not heart disease or cancer. What else do people voluntarily accept that carries a risk of dying at the rate of one in 50?

As a clinician–scientist, driven by the painful but still fresh recollection of Tom Martin's death, I felt compelled to try to attack this problem—the ultimate complication of total hip replacement surgery.

In the interim between Tom Martin's death and the introduction of total hip surgery in the United States, I had already shown that I could reduce the incidence of blood clots forming in the leg in older patients who had sustained a hip fracture by using a blood thinner called Warfarin. Now, in 1969, as we began our own experience with total hip replacements in the United States, for the very first time, I applied this "outrageous" approach to total hip arthroplasty. Although it was widely thought to be "outrageous" because it was clearly counterintuitive to use a blood thinner in conjunction with major hip surgery, it worked. It worked despite an increased risk of bleeding in the wound. Indeed, this blood thinner is still used today, nearly 50 years later.

Subsequently, during the early 1970s, I introduced for the first time another agent—ordinary aspirin—as an agent for the prophylaxis against fatal pulmonary emboli, which is now increasingly and widely used around the world for just this purpose. Throughout the succeeding years, many other forms of prophylaxis were also introduced successfully. In short, because of the success of these new preventative measures, the risk of a fatal pulmonary embolus following total hip replacement has plummeted from the devastating figure of one in 50 patients by more than an order of magnitude: to the very low level of one in 1000. And in my own practice I was able to do more than 3000 consecutive total hip replacements without a single fatal pulmonary embolus.

I mention this remarkable improvement—in decreasing the extremely high risk of fatal pulmonary embolization following total hip replacement surgery in the early years—to introduce a virtual revolution that took place during the first five decades of total hip surgery to control aggressively or even eliminate completely these high dangers that existed when total hip replacement was first performed.

Nearly all of the severe complications that plagued total hip replacement surgery during the early 1960s have been overcome.

The breaking of stems does not occur any more. Infection is now at the 0.5% level. Fixing of the thigh piece to the femur is virtually universally successful. So, too, is fixing the socket piece to the pelvis. Dislocation has been remarkably reduced and, as mentioned, fatal pulmonary embolism has been strikingly reduced.

All these complications were reduced by about a factor of 10 or more. *Except for one.*

The severe bone destruction we first saw in Peter Dunn and the three companion cases was not only startling, but at that time was considered exceedingly rare, bizarre, and unexplained, and was even unnamed. But, instead of being reduced, like all these other severe complications I have just mentioned, this strange bone destruction simply increased and increased and increased. It became far more widely observed, and then far more widely feared. As it progressively increased in frequency, it led to more and more reoperations. And then to more and more complex and difficult reoperations. The additional frequency and severity of this bone destruction radically altered the daily practice of total hip surgery.

This bone destruction adjacent to the prosthesis, which appeared at first to be a rare, bizarre, ill-defined, and unnamed complication, went in exactly the opposite direction of all the other major complications of the operation. It became the single most frequent and single most important late complication in all of total hip replacement surgery.

It became, over time, the leading cause of pain after total hip replacement, the leading cause of thigh pieces becoming loose from the bone, the leading cause of socket components coming loose from the bone, the leading cause of fractures of the femur, the leading cause of fractures of the pelvis, and, most critically, the leading cause of reoperation after total hip replacement. At its peak, it affected an estimated one million patients or more.

Thus it was that this striking but exceedingly mysterious bone destruction adjacent to the prostheses ultimately became the number-one enemy of successful total hip replacement. What to do?

Chapter 4

The First Real Breakthrough

*Research consists in seeing what everyone else has seen,
but thinking what no one else has thought.*

—ALBERT SZENT-GYORGYI, *Nobel laureate,*
the first to identify vitamin C

In her early 40s, Miranda Clarke began to struggle to get out of bed in the morning. No matter how much she slept, she woke fatigued. Her joints became so stiff she had to lean on the night-stand and roll up onto her feet. This was a painful contortion, but she never complained. Miranda did not like to let things get her down.

Getting through the day became a challenge. Her kids were old enough to have busy after-school schedules, yet they were not old enough to drive. She was glad to take them to their soccer games and piano lessons, but every moment she sat behind the wheel was agony. Despite her strong resolve, she sometimes gave way to tears after she dropped them off. How could she see them through high school, and college after that, if this pain kept getting worse?

Her doctor had diagnosed her with rheumatoid arthritis, and when he eventually recommended a cup arthroplasty—the only hip reconstruction available for rheumatoid arthritis at that time—Miranda readily agreed. The surgery gave her greater mobility at first. She could drive her kids around without suffering, but she could not, even then, join them on weekend bike rides in the park. Her reprieve didn't last very long. In two years, she had to have a repeat cup arthroplasty; but, by the time it had become clear that this second reconstruction helped even less, total hip operations had been approved by the Food and Drug Administration (FDA) for use in the United States. So, Miranda had a total hip replacement.

One day in 1980, seven years after her total hip replacement, while she was shopping with a friend, a sharp pain shot through her leg like a bolt of lightning and she collapsed on the floor. Her femur had snapped.

An ambulance rushed her to the hospital. She was confined to bed with her right leg suspended in a full-length leg sling. The fracture was so obvious on the x-ray that a premedical student would have seen it. What alarmed her surgeon even more than the femur fracture was the extensive destruction of the bone around the hip, both in her femur and her socket (Figures 4.1 and 4.2). Because of this bone destruction, the femur had shattered into multiple large and small fragments, and the pelvic bone had been so eroded the entire artificial socket was loose. Her surgeon phoned me and asked whether I could help with this complex reconstruction crisis.

The first problem was the fragmentation of the femur. Somehow, I needed to replace completely the upper half of her thigh bone. There was no easy way to do this. Among the two daunting possible options, we could either use a huge metal prosthesis to replace the upper half of her femur or replace the upper half of her femur with a corresponding segment of a femur from the bone bank.

After that, ideally, we would redo her total hip replacement, but Miranda's pelvic bone was so severely eroded from the three prior hip operations plus—you guessed it—bone destruction around the prosthesis, we could not simply insert another total

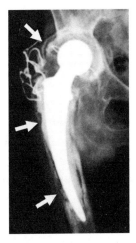

FIGURE 4.1 *Bone Destruction of Femur and Pelvis*

X-ray of the front view of the right hip showing a total hip replacement with major bone destruction in both the femur and the pelvis. Reprinted with permission and copyright © of the British Editorial Society of Bone and Joint Surgery from Mulroy, RD, Mankin, HJ, Harris WH. Insertion of a prosthetic hip into a total hip allograft: case report. *J Bone Joint Surg [Br]* 1990;72-B:643–646, figures 1a and 1b.

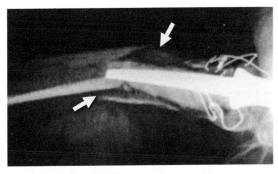

FIGURE 4.2 *Femur Snapped (Side View)*

X-ray of a side view of the same femur showing that the femur snapped. Reprinted with permission and copyright © of the British Editorial Society of Bone and Joint Surgery from Mulroy, RD, Mankin, HJ, Harris WH. Insertion of a prosthetic hip into a total hip allograft: case report. *J Bone Joint Surg [Br]* 1990;72-B:643–646, figures 1a and 1b.

hip socket. We, somehow, had to add a bone graft to restore the pelvic bone enough to redo the hip socket. This same mysterious disease process that had aggressively destroyed her femur to the point that it snapped while she was simply walking had also made the socket piece completely loose. Although the mystery of the bone destruction continued to plague me, I had to turn my attention to solving the problem at hand.

What Miranda needed was a "fresh start." And this required fresh thinking. What if we could find a portion of pelvic bone in the bone bank to replace the hip socket area and then also replace the upper end of the femur with bone from the bone bank? We would, in effect, replace the entire hip joint with intact bony structures from the bone bank. Moreover, if the femur and the pelvic bone were from the same donor, we would be inserting a perfectly matched hip pair.

This would not be a hip replacement, but a *hip transplant*. And it had never been done before.

It was essential to obtain the bone bank femur and bone bank socket from the same donor so that the ball of the femur would fit perfectly into its natural socket; otherwise, the mismatched joint would wear out rapidly. In addition, there were other long-term complications such as rejection, fracture, and late infection that might arise from such a massive hip transplant, but Miranda readily agreed to assume these risks with us. Her immediate problem was so dire that this radical proposal was by far the best chance she had.

The operation was complex, long, difficult, and demanding, but it was a complete success. In a marvelous reflection of what a positive and resilient person she was, Miranda greeted us the next morning with a smile—wearing lipstick! For a patient to put on lipstick the day after such a long and complex operation is exceedingly rare and a clear manifestation of both her striking resilience and her determination to get back to normal.

During her rehabilitation, she passed two vital landmarks. She became able to walk pain free on her hip transplant using only one crutch. Simultaneously, the bone was beautifully restored in both her femur and pelvis. And, in fact, she had the best seven years of her life since the rheumatoid arthritis had first crippled her.

Toward the end of those seven good years, the ball of the transplanted femur began to fail. This was one of the risks we had all faced together, knowing the transplanted ball would not have any direct blood supply, and therefore was at risk of collapse over time. When it did collapse seven years later, we gave Miranda a second total hip replacement. But, *this* total hip replacement inserted directly into her hip transplant, just as we'd planned. And she was back in business.

Miranda's case was extremely severe. No one else ever had to endure two of the old-type hip reconstructions followed by a total hip replacement, and then a full hip transplant followed by one more total hip! But, as we knew from the x-rays, and as the pathology of the tissue from the broken femur and the loose socket confirmed, the source of Miranda's suffering was the same strange, nonmalignant, noninfectious bone destruction we'd first seen in Peter Dunn.

Increasingly, this mysterious disease, which had appeared to be so rare at first, became the dominant cause of failure of total hip replacement and the single most common reason for reoperations. Ironically, few patients and even fewer people in the general population even knew the name of this process. Both to the patients, and even more so to the general population, it was a disease without a name. Why was that?

As the increasing incidence of the bone destruction became more widely recognized and the disease became somewhat better understood, it was, unfortunately, given the jaw-breaking medical name of *periprosthetic osteolysis.* The name itself is quite revealing in Latin: *peri* ("in the area of"), prosthetic ("prosthesis"), *osteo* ("bone"), *lysis* ("destruction"), or "bone destruction in the area of the prosthesis," but few people speak Latin. Because the disease was totally new, enigmatic, and confusing at the time, its name never became a household phrase like diabetes or cancer.

Even after the research on this disease became more widely known, few surgeons chose to share its name or the complexities of its molecular biology with their patients. Instead, when surgeons made the diagnosis, they had the choice of explaining the complexities of this totally new disease or, far more simply, they could say: "Unfortunately, the bone has broken. It looks like we'll need to operate." Most surgeons and, in fact, most patients preferred the latter. For most patients, when they knew they needed another operation because the prosthesis had come loose or the bone had fractured, to know the details about a strange and obscure disease called *periprosthetic osteolysis* was an unnecessary overload. That is why, both then and even now, few patients (and even fewer among the general public) have ever heard of the official term for this common worldwide disease.

Despite its molecular complexity and unwieldy name, periprosthetic osteolysis, a stealth disease, became the leading "silent killer" of those exceptional expectations of total hip replacements.

At about the time of our publication of the four cases in 1976, the first real breakthrough occurred in developing a fresh and exciting concept of what in the world might be causing this bone destruction. Dr. Hans Willert developed his seminal theory regarding this aggressive bone destruction (Profile 4.1).

Using special histological techniques, Willert was able to demonstrate that there were tiny particles of the plastic substance commonly called "bone cement" *inside* the macrophages in the tissue in the areas where the bone destruction occurred. Bone cement acts like putty, and it is used to affix the artificial

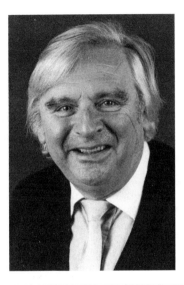

Reproduced with permission of Prof. Dr. med. Gorg Koster, Schön Klinik, Schön Klinik Lorsch, Lorsch, Germany

Hans Willert (1934–2006) had a fascinating and unusual life. He was born in Greiz, Thuringen, Germany, and received his medical degree from the University of Leipzig, East Germany. Trapped in East Germany as a young man after the erection of the Berlin Wall, with the consent of his family he fled to West Germany.

How do you circumvent the Berlin Wall? One stop on the East Berlin underground approached West Berlin near the Brandenburg gate. He entered the underground near his home, carrying only his violin, as he often did while going to his weekly violin lesson. On that day, as the underground approached West Berlin, he fled to West Berlin. Many died attempting to escape from East Berlin, but Willert was successful, taking with him nothing but his violin. It would be another 20 years before the Berlin Wall fell. Had he waited, medical science would have lost the benefit of his unique insights.

With his freedom restored, Willert furthered his education in medicine by completing nine years of study in pathology with an emphasis on bone pathology, an additional experience that ultimately proved uniquely valuable. His orthopaedic training began late, in 1969, at the University of Frankfurt/Main. He then was appointed head of bone diseases in the orthopaedic hospital in Frankfurt and subsequently became chief of the orthopaedic clinic at Georg-August University in Gottingen, Germany.

It was through his training as a pathologist that his mind was oriented to ponder the mysterious process of this bone destruction from the specific point of view of the type of cells and type of cellular reactions that might be causing it. This led to his key observation that the ingestion of tiny particles of bone cement into the macrophages themselves was the underlying mechanism for the stimulation of the macrophages and thus, ultimately, for the destruction of bone. Bone cement is the plastic grouting material that Charnley introduced to hold the artificial parts of the total hip rigidly to the skeleton (see more about bone cement later in this chapter).

components of total hip replacements to the skeleton. For example, in the thigh bone (or femur) the bone cement is inserted down the narrow cavity of the femur. The thigh piece of the total hip implant is then forced into the putty. Then, in about 10 minutes or so, the bone cement changes its characteristics to become completely hard, locking the thigh piece rigidly to the bone.

This remarkable observation of finding tiny particles of bone cement inside the macrophages validated Willert's striking explanation for this disturbing bone destruction—namely, that it was caused by the stimulation of the body's natural defense cells (macrophages) by the ingestion of tiny particles of bone cement into those cells.

Willert postulated that the ingestion of the particles of bone cement by macrophages was the underlying mechanism that caused the bone destruction. When the macrophages began to do their job, by ingesting the foreign material in the body, the tiny particles of bone cement stimulated an overproduction of additional macrophages, which then, somehow, resulted in the devastating erosion of the bone. Although Willert's insightful idea seemed to explain the strange "sheets of macrophages" we observed in Peter Dunn's biopsy, something still bothered me. Even if it were true that the cement particles were stimulating macrophages, that didn't change the fact that macrophages cannot resorb bone. Many other diseases involve the ingestion of small particles by macrophages, but none of them lead to resorption of bone.

How could even a large number of macrophages result in bone destruction? Willert's imaginative theory left that critical question completely unanswered, and that wasn't the only problem. As the number of total hip replacements increased, new problems began to emerge.

In x-rays of patients with hip replacements that were 10 years old or more, surgeons began to notice a dark zone between the bone cement around the hip socket component and the adjacent bone. It was named *demarcation,* and the implications were clear. The bone in the pelvis that was immediately adjacent to the bone cement was also being carved away.

To make matters worse, Charnley found that by 10 to 12 years after a total hip replacement, demarcation was quite common— present in 59% of all hip replacements. Furthermore, his research revealed the demarcation was extensive in 25% of cases. Among that group, for half of those patients, the entire socket component had come completely loose from the pelvis and moved to a new position.

How did these utterly different phenomena—demarcation and migration of the socket component—relate to the destruction of bone in the femur, called *cavitation,* as if a cavity had occurred in the femur? Were these three processes identical, different, or unrelated?

In science, we are generally urged to attempt to find a single explanation rather than multiple, complex explanations for any unknown phenomenon, at least at first. These new observations added substantially to our quandary.

All the while, as we were wondering what to make of the increasing frequency of this bone-destroying disease, surgeons around the world were removing patients' failed total hips and installing new total hip replacements in their place, knowing that it was only a matter of time before some of these new hip replacements would need to be replaced yet again *for the same reason.* We were quickly realizing that *reoperations,* or *revisions,* as they are also called, were far more complex than the initial surgery—with far less satisfactory results.

Ironically, in many instances these "revisions" were far more complex specifically because of the very bone destruction that made them necessary. This extensive loss of bone often mandated the use of massive bone grafting during these revision operations, which was more demanding on both the patient and the surgeon, and required far more time on the operating table. The risk of infection and death was higher as well. How could we, as orthopaedic surgeons, continue to recommend total hip surgery so readily when it was becoming, progressively, an operation that was likely to fail for one quarter to one third of our patients? With hundreds of thousands of existing hip replacements hovering in a netherworld between magnificent success and impending failure, the clock was ticking.

Willert's explanation of the ingestion of particles of bone cement by the macrophages remained, by far, the most substantial hypothesis. Increasing evidence supported his proposal, despite the fact that the concept was additionally challenged by some specific studies of the bone resorption around some of the loose socket pieces that did not show any fragmentation of the bone cement.

Over time, surgeons began to see increasing numbers of patients whose bone cement had fatigued and was breaking into small fragments. This fragmentation only accelerated the ingestion of fragmented bone cement by macrophages. If Willert was right, it should have accelerated bone destruction as well. It did.

Ever since *Clinical Orthopaedics and Related Research*, a leading, peer-reviewed orthopaedic journal, published an important article by Lynn Jones and David Hungerford called "Cement Disease" in 1987, this report has been widely quoted as evidence that the bone destruction was truly a disease caused by the cement particles.

Intent as I was to find the explanation, I couldn't ignore the fact that the concept of cement disease left unresolved two key questions. First, how does the stimulation of macrophages induce bone resorption, because macrophages cannot resorb bone? Second, what caused the bone destruction in cases that showed no fragmented bone cement? The need to find a solution was urgent, with or without an explanation for these two critical questions.

The obvious way to solve the problem of cement disease was to eliminate the use of bone cement altogether. Fortunately, groups of innovators had been working quietly on a "cement-less" form of total hip arthroplasty for a number of years. The basic concept behind cementless total hip fixation to the skeleton is to have bone grow directly into the total hip components themselves, locking the compound to the skeleton. The most promising concept for this consisted of a layer of metal that had pores in it (the porous layer) on the outer surface of the metal implant. If the patient's own bone could be induced to grow directly into that porous layer, fixing the components to the skeleton, no bone cement was needed. Ergo, there could be no cement disease.

Outstanding among the many capable contributors to this remarkable progression in total hip replacement—namely, the development of cementless total hip implants—were Jorge Galante and his coworker William Rostocker at Rush Medical School, and Canadian materials scientist Bob Pillier along with his devotees Charles Engh and Robert Kenna.

In many quarters of the world, the new "cementless" total hip replacements swept the field as soon as the designs were perfected. After decades of uncertainty and some very disappointing outcomes using some of the early cementless designs, a great feeling of calm spread happily across the field of hip surgery. With the wide acceptance of the concept of cement disease, the problem of bone destruction appeared to have been solved simply by eliminating the use of bone cement by virtue of "going cementless." It looked like we were back in business.

Except we were wrong.

Chapter 5

Meanwhile, Back at the Ranch . . .

No great discovery is ever made without a bold guess.
—ISAAC NEWTON

As the relentless search to find the cause of the terrible bone destruction adjacent to prostheses continued, it remained important that we persisted in making strides in completely new applications of total hip replacement surgery. And yet, the sword of bone resorption hung over our efforts. And so it was that during the 1970s I created other vital development in total hip surgery that, although not specifically related to the bone destruction problem, was also subject to it in the long run.

As the dramatic results of the successful total hip replacements prompted speculations on innovative solutions to other currently untreatable hip joint conditions, the most challenging of these was severe arthritis of the hip in the adult because of total dislocation of the hip at birth. A solution to this extreme problem had never been found. But even if some kind of an unique total hip replacement were developed in an attempt to solve this issue, it, too, ran the risk of the bone destruction disease.

Because I'd come to know and respect John Charnley during my ABC Traveling Fellowship in Orthopaedics in the United Kingdom, I was especially intrigued when he, the originator of total hip replacement, declared that one procedure was beyond the scope of total hip replacements—this very problem of arthritis of the hip in the adult patient because of total dislocation of the hip at birth. So this represented a challenge.

A number of children are born with an underdeveloped hip socket. If the abnormality is severe enough, the ball of their hip lies completely outside the socket. To make matters worse, the same circumstances that cause the malformed hip socket also can result in extraordinary abnormalities of the upper part of the thigh bone. Girls are prone to this condition far more than boys by 20 to one.

Surprisingly enough, as these patients grow older, pain is not their biggest problem. In fact, some people with this condition suffer no pain until relatively late in life. But throughout their lives, they are unable walk without a very bad limp. Because the condition commonly affects both hips, they have a very unattractive characteristic waddling gait.

When Gina Holstead came into my office, her limp was already very severe. She had been born with a complete dislocation of the ball of the femur out of the hip socket on each side. Gina had learned to compensate by wrenching her shoulders side-to-side as she walked, throughout all her life. I marveled that her situation had not caused her perpetual pain much sooner.

At 48 years old, Gina started to experience pain. By the time I saw her two years later, she had a serious disability. At that time, she was using two canes because of the pain, which had come on progressively. Even with strong pain medicine, her life was at a full stop.

Compounding the problem was the fact that Gina had been born with an endocrine disease characterized by a complete lack of estrogens. As a result, she had only grown to 4 feet 8 inches tall. Still, until the pain took hold, she had made an admirable adjustment to this unusual and severe combination of endocrine and orthopaedic abnormalities.

Creating a surgical solution for this problem of complete dislocation of the hips from birth had no precedent. It meant creating unique, untested implants and generating completely new techniques of inserting them. Together, she and I faced several challenging problems. None of these problems had ever been addressed before.

- **Severely underdeveloped pelvis.** Because her pelvis was extremely underdeveloped, no existing artificial socket would fit (Figure 5.1).
- **Undersized femur.** Her thigh bone was so tiny that no existing thigh component would fit.
- **Dislocated femur head.** The ball of her femur was in the wrong place—completely above the socket. Somehow, we would have to bring the femur down so that the artificial ball would fit into the newly reconstructed hip socket that we would have to create.
- **Shortened muscles and nerves with distorted arteries.** Her hip muscles were so short they prevented us from pulling the femur down far enough to fit into the reconstructed hip socket. The nerves and the muscles did not lie in their normal positions.

Some years before, I invented the technique of adding a bone graft to increase the bone volume of the pelvis at the hip socket for patients with moderately compromised hip sockets. So I started with the idea of adding bone to Gina's very tiny hip socket. If the bone I used to augment her shallow hip socket was the bone of the ball of her own femur, which I would otherwise discard, there would be no problem of bone rejection or incompatibility.

Even with that, however, conventional implants would be much too large for Gina. My only choice was to design a very

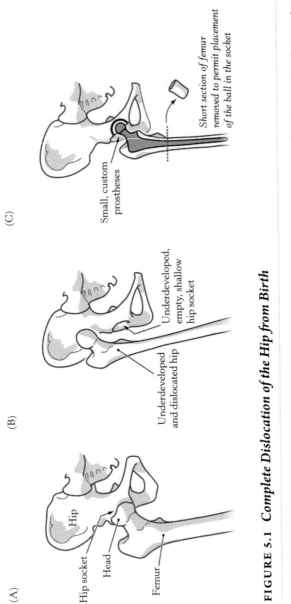

(A)

(B)

(C)

Hip socket

Hip

Head

Femur

Underdeveloped
and dislocated hip

Underdeveloped,
empty, shallow
hip socket

Small, custom
prostheses

Short section of femur
removed to permit placement
of the ball in the socket

FIGURE 5.1 *Complete Dislocation of the Hip from Birth*

(A) Normal hip anatomy. (B) Developmental total dislocation of the hip. (C) Surgical repair (total hip arthroplasty with shortening of the femur). Printed with permission from Cassio Lynm, manager of Amino Creative, LLC, Stoneham, MA.

small artificial hip socket and a very tiny thigh piece with an extremely small ball. The entire implant would have to be much smaller than anything that had ever been used before. The artificial hip socket would be, instead of about one half the size of an orange, *about the size of a thimble!*

The emotional landscape surrounding the formulation of innovation in surgical capability is complex. The desire to achieve a distinctly positive outcome for the patient is blended with apprehension, not quite fear, both about creating harm rather than good and about failure even if distinct harm does not occur. All the uncertainty of an untried venture abounds, particularly because the "experiment" is on a fellow human being. Still, one is driven by the pain, suffering, and compromises in the life of that individual, so the urge to proceed is strong. One is also abetted by successful experiences of prior smaller steps, which could increase the likelihood of success. I had been successful previously in augmenting the amount of pelvic bone available for a total hip operation by originating the idea of adding large bone grafts such as the ball of the hip joint, which is ordinarily discarded. I knew that concept might help Gina as well.

As I began to address the problem of the shortened muscles, a new idea occurred to me that was pivotal to the success of the entire procedure. I suddenly realized that if I cut off the ball from her femur and removed the gristle that surrounds the hip joint, called the *hip capsule,* I could slowly and gently pull the femur down by putting her leg in traction for several weeks after the operation. And the ball of the femur could be used later for the bone graft itself.

This preliminary operation would also allow me to measure precisely the size of her hip socket, so I'd know exactly how large to make the artificial hip socket I was building. All this work, of course, occurred long before the invention of the very special x-ray technique of computed tomography or CT, which, in today's world, would have let me know the dimensions of the femur and the hip socket just from the x-ray scan itself.

With the success of these procedures being critically dependent on so many innovations, I had numerous, thorough discussions with Gina and her family about the risks. I explained that nothing like this had ever been attempted before. I wanted all of us to have a clear understanding that it might not work. Despite the unknowns, Gina was fully committed to go forward because of her disabling pain.

To our mutual delight, the two operations went surprisingly well and she experienced no adverse effects afterward. I then proceeded to reconstruct her other hip as well. Her extraordinarily unusual problem had forced us into an entirely new realm. We now knew how to do total hip reconstructions on patients whose ball had never been in the hip socket from birth.

Another patient I encountered with disabling pain from the same condition (total dislocation of the hip from birth) was complicated by yet a different disease, Down syndrome, with substantial mental retardation. At five feet, Margaret Reardon was just slightly taller than Gina. Yet, we faced similar challenges because her skeleton was also so small that ordinary components would not fit. Having made such tiny devices for Gina, it was feasible that we could do the same thing for Margaret. A very small, custom-made femoral component with an equally small ball was likely to be effective.

If Margaret was unfortunate in the limitations imposed on her by Down syndrome, she was extremely fortunate in the enormity of compassion and dedication she received from her parents and two brothers. Even after their parents died, her two older brothers stood by her side. Margaret was happy, active, and responsible within the loving confines of their close supervision.

My only hesitation was that a total hip replacement patient must observe certain restrictions about the positions and motions of her leg after surgery to prevent the hip from dislocating. With Margaret's limited capacity for comprehension, I had concerns she would not be able to abide by these crucial limitations. After several discussions with her brothers, and after obtaining their consent in addition to hers to proceed, I became convinced their extraordinary devotion to her would allow us to do a total hip replacement and probably manage her course successfully thereafter. No other operation would begin to provide her with the same level of function and relief of pain.

Margaret's problem was unusual. The number of patients with Down syndrome who require a total hip—and especially one this tiny—is, indeed, small. The overwhelming majority of all total hip patients are full-size, competent adults older than 50 years. And yet, the emotional return to the patient, to the family, and, not incidentally, to the surgeon and the surgical team, is outsized in instances such as these, in which the possibility of a good outcome can be offered in types of cases that previously were beyond the pale. Yet, these expectations carry higher risks.

The operation went well, and the plan nearly worked out as we had hoped. Then, Margaret dislocated her hip.

With such a tiny ball, dislocation had always been one of the major risks. With a normal-size implant and a patient who could maintain the right precautions, I would have simply put the hip back into position and given the patient a brace to limit motion while it healed. But Margaret was upset by the brace. After exploring that possibility, we all realized it was not likely to work.

The alternative was a difficult one. After returning the hip to its correct position, we had to put this wonderful young lady into a full-body cast for six weeks—from the tip of her right toes up to her armpits and down to her left knee. This dramatically increased the level of caretaking required by her brothers, but they did it willingly and reaped the rewards.

When Margaret came out of the cast with her hip fully healed, her exuberance was uncontained. She was thrilled to be free from "that awful cast," and the pain relief enabled her to resume her usual activities with the devoted siblings she loved.

It is gratifying to say that operations such as these on patients with congenital hip dislocations in which the ball is totally out of the socket are now common all around the world using these techniques. Not only did this extension of the applications of total hip replacements allow me to help people who had always, up until that time, been considered untreatable, but also it increased the determination I had to find a solution to the bone destruction problem because these types of cases cannot be approached by any other operation except a total hip prosthesis, even as severely modified as they are. That meant these patients would also be at risk for the severe bone destruction, as were all other total hip patients.

Chapter 6

Is It Really Cement Disease?

The most exciting phrase to hear in science, the one that heralds new discoveries, is not "Eureka!" but "That's funny...."

—ISAAC ASIMOV

Final preparations just before leaving to attend any scientific meeting, particularly if your work has been accepted for presentation to your peers, are always hectic. All the data upon which the presentation is based must be rechecked for validity and accuracy. Usually, there is a last-minute rush to finish the preparation of the slides to include the latest information or to generate the most relevant and dramatic conclusions. It's an exciting, stress-filled rush—even more so if your presentation promotes controversy, which is, of course, the nature of good science.

The other factor that increases the routine anxiety of such a trip is what I call the *grieving of leaving.* "Grieving" may be too strong a word, but there are natural regrets every time you go away. As a clinician, it is always a challenge to leave patients who are not progressing as well as you would prefer, or perhaps there are family problems, political issues, or personal issues. As a scientist, I am always in the middle of experiments that must, regrettably, be suspended until I return.

It was September 1989. I was preparing to fly to Montreal for a meeting of the Hip Society, a group of North American leaders in hip surgery specifically selected because of the innovations and advancements they have contributed to the field. Because I had been the first president of the Hip Society, I was particularly eager for my presentation to go well, but my enthusiasm was also stoked because we had some innovative ideas to share.

My last activity before leaving was to conduct a routine review of all the x-rays of all my patients with the new cementless total hip replacement I had designed with Jorge Galante, Professor and Chief of Orthopaedic Surgery, Rush Medical College, Chicago, Illinois. At least I thought it was routine. Disaster struck in the form of periprosthetic osteolysis!

There it was. Classical and pure. Localized bone destruction of the femur exactly like the cavitation of cement disease—without the cement! How could that be? What would it do to our cherished hypothesis about *cement* actually causing cement disease?

Defensively, I mused, "Well, . . . it's just one case." But, as our stunned review continued, there was a second, then a third within the first 100 cases alone. This meant a 3% incidence of yet another problem we had never seen in all the prior reviews of our cementless total hip replacements.

We rechecked everything. There was no mix-up. Yet again we were faced with an inexplicable phenomenon. Was this a different disease or had our original theory been completely wrong?

After flying to Montreal that evening, I reached Dr. Galante in Chicago by phone Saturday morning. He was startled and appalled by my news, but took immediate action. He called his research team to the laboratory Saturday morning to submit the x-rays of his own patients to the same "routine" review that I had done. Not only was his process the same as mine, so, too, were his results: bone destruction in cementless total hip replacements at a rate of 3%.

This was striking information. It meant this disturbing form of bone destruction was independent of whether cement was used and therefore had to be the result of one or more entirely independent causes.

At the Hip Society meeting that afternoon, I announced this finding to a stunned audience of mystified and perplexed hip surgeons. With one exception, no one else had seen anything like this. John Callaghan an outstanding orthopaedic surgeon at the University of Iowa, had seen *one* similar instance.

This one instance proved to be of great importance, because it quickly narrowed the variables. Our implants had been manufactured by Zimmer using a metal called *titanium*, with a porous surface called *fibermetal*. Callaghan's implant had been manufactured by a different company, Howmedica, using a different metal, chrome cobalt, with a different porous surface made of *chrome cobalt beads*. This meant the destruction was *not* limited to implants made by just one company, one metal type, or one type of porous surface. Instantly, Dr. Callaghan's single similar but distinctly different example saved us from three blind avenues of research, but the mystery remained.

It was time to go back to the drawing board. Clearly there was cement disease, but what in the world was this, in the complete absence of bone cement? What could it be?

As more of these types of cases were recognized—and then in some cases tissue was examined under the microscope—in case after case, the biopsies of bone destruction in cases of cementless total hip replacements showed *exactly the same characteristics* I had seen initially in the biopsy from Peter Dunn: "sheets of macrophages and aggressive bone resorption," along with the complete absence of infection.

When we published the first article showing that this bone destruction could occur in patients with cementless total hip prostheses in 1990, it was a full 14 years after we published the four mysterious cases of bone destruction in cases of cemented total hips. We reported that the basic characteristics of the disease were exactly the same—*with or without cement.* Moreover, as more time passed, it became clear that the incidence of the bone destruction, the severity of the bone destruction, the spontaneous fractures, and the loose prostheses all increased progressively with both types of prostheses. Eventually, in both types, the prostheses forced between 15% to 40% of patients to undergo revision operations. As before, these revision operations were more complex than the primary operations, and they had far worse outcomes. They were more likely to get infected and, alas, were more likely to be fatal. In fact, in certain designs of cementless total hip prostheses, the incidence of bone destruction was actually worse than with a cemented prosthesis.

Although bone destruction was occurring in at least 20% of all patients in many series—and in some series as high as 40%— for young patients whose vigor and activity put them most at risk, with one design it was an astonishing 60%! And for all those patients who developed bone destruction after surgery, the "miraculous" results of a total hip replacement became a haunting illusion.

In science, it is often true that what seems to be a rare observation, an outlier against the conventional wisdom, ultimately forces a reevaluation of the fundamental question. This was exactly such a case. In laboratories and Grand Rounds across the world, surgeons were actively assessing all their basic assumptions and asking new questions.

Some of our initial questions about cement disease resurfaced as well: Without bone cement present, what in the world could be causing bone resorption? Why were the macrophages forming those peculiar sheets? After all, cementless implants had been created to solve the problem of bone destruction around implants that required cement.

Naturally, many theories arose. Some speculated the large porous surface area in the cementless implants was causing some kind of an adverse reaction. Others focused their attention on the "press-fit" technique used to insert cementless components. Using the press-fit technique, components were wedged judiciously, but forcibly, into a hole in the bone slightly smaller than the implant itself, literally jammed in place for a tight fit. Was this causing a bone resorption reaction? A huge effort was directed toward solving this fresh enigma.

When we finally solved this conundrum, the answer was astonishing beyond belief. Willert's *general* concept had been right all along!

The macrophages were, indeed, ingesting small particles of foreign material, as he had suggested. But in this case, it was not the cement particles that were attracting and stimulating the macrophages. The entirely new and unexpected observation was that small particles of the *polyethylene*, the plastic that replaced the worn cartilage in the hip socket, were the culprit.

Over time, motion at the hip joint wore off tiny particles of the polyethylene, which were gobbled up by the body's defense cells, the *macrophages*, just as we found earlier with cement particles. This wear was low—much slower than in Charnley's PTFE—so low that it had been completely discounted.

Intense productivity from many outstanding centers, including John Charnley in Great Britain, the Mayo Clinic led by Mark Coventry, the University of California Los Angeles (UCLA) under Harlan Amstutz, the Hospital for Special Surgery chaired by Philip D. Wilson, Jr., and many other creative European institutions, showed that the greatest culprit was not cement particles, but polyethylene particles. The term *cement disease* had been correct in part, but stopped short of recognizing this aspect of the problem. Tiny particles of bone cement could and did lead to stimulation of macrophages, and thus ultimately to the resorption of bone. Because we now knew that particles of both bone cement *and* polyethylene were equally capable of being the stimulating agent, the more accurate diagnosis and the only inclusive diagnosis was *particle disease.*

Because Charnley's new polyethylene had appeared for many years to be so wonderfully durable, it surprised all of us that polyethylene was part of the problem. Even more puzzling, in all the many other uses of this specific polyethylene in industry, wear of this polyethylene produced big chunks of polyethylene, not the tiny particles small enough to get the macrophages' attention and be ingested by them.

For either a polyethylene or a cement particle to be small enough to be eaten by a macrophage, it has to be about one micron or smaller. That's extremely small—1/25,000th of an inch. A tiny grain of sand is 100 microns. Many human hairs are about 100 microns in width. A micron is smaller than anything you can see. A single particle of smoke from a cigarette is smaller than one micron. Most of the particles leading to the macrophage response, and thus to the bone damage, were even smaller—what we call *submicron*—in diameter.

So, this raised yet another unanswered query. What was so special about the specific circumstances of the use of polyethylene in total hips that made the wear process generate such miniscule particles?

The arresting dichotomy was this: The striking and rejuvenating success for so many total hip patients contrasted acutely with the fate of those who got the serious bone destruction who were at high risk—with even for some, their lives on the line. Exhaustive research was sharply focused on this very question. Strangely enough, in many cases there was relatively little apparent wear of the polyethylene—far less than with Charnley's PTFE—but the actual numbers of particles released were huge. In fact, one estimate was that with each step, seven *billion* particles were released!

Total hip surgery, for all of its recognized majesty, had unwittingly and simultaneously produced in the body an *internal particle generator*, a device buried deep in the human body that generated submicron particles of plastic in high numbers on a daily basis. Because the average person takes nearly two million steps per year, each device might well generate almost a trillion particles during its life span.

An urgent, massive scientific investigation wasn't just needed, it was demanded. One key mystery was the same one that had been with us from the start: How did the ingestion of tiny particles by macrophages lead to bone destruction? The recognition of bone destruction in cementless total hips during the early '90s added a new one: What makes wear of the polyethylene, only in the circumstances of human gait, generate submicron particles?

The ultimate mechanism by which bone gets removed is not a mystery; it is obvious. Because only osteoclasts can remove bone, the agent of removal had to be the osteoclasts. But the total unknown was: How do *they* get involved? The solution to this question hinged on our ability to unravel the molecular biology of this strange disease.

One of the great joys of being at the MGH is the enormous breadth of the research activities that are constantly in motion. During the early 1980s, while we were still under the impression that cement particles were the sole instigator of the bone destruction, the arthritis unit at the MGH was involved in a vibrant research endeavor investigating the basic molecular biology of rheumatoid arthritis. It seemed highly likely to me that the very techniques being used for that purpose might have a direct application to the mystery I was trying to unravel.

What I needed was a resourceful partner with a high level of those very specific skills to launch the investigation into particle disease. Steve Goldring of the arthritis unit was just the man. Steve's early work had helped establish a critical aspect of the role that osteoclasts play in bone destruction. This made him an ideal collaborator for this investigation (Profile 6.1). For the microscopic analysis, I recruited Andy Rosenberg of the pathology department. We were the first to attack the molecular biology of this strange disease.

Because the MGH is a major referral center for the revision operations on patients with failed hip replacement, plus my compelling interest in eliminating this disease of aggressive bone destruction, I had both the opportunity and the passion to spend many days—and not a few nights—operating on some of the most severe cases of bone destruction. Ubiquitous in every one of these operations was the need to strip away that layer of soft fibrous tissue from the bone adjacent to the worst bone destruction. Typically, surgeons commonly discarded this tissue or perhaps sent it to the pathologist for microscopic analysis. No one had bothered to study it from the point of view of its biological activity.

Thus it was that when we examined this tissue in Steve's lab, we found the first step toward the answer to the question that had been plaguing me since the first time I'd seen it in Peter Dunn: What was causing the massive bone destruction around the hip prostheses? Hans Willert had made the singularly important stride by drawing attention to the fact that macrophages were ingesting tiny particles. Later on, during the 1990s, subsequent research had expanded his insights to include the tiny polyethylene particles. But, one stubborn fact remained: No matter what

PROFILE 6.1 Steven Goldring, MD

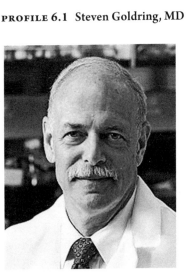

Image courtesy of and reprinted with permission by Dr. S. Goldring.

Dr. Steven Goldring is a clinician–scientist, one of that uncommon breed who works in the interdisciplinary space that incorporates both medicine and biological science. Although initially trained as a rheumatologist, he later became the chief *scientific* officer at one of the nation's premiere orthopaedic institutions: the Hospital for Special Surgery in New York City.

A graduate of Williams College and Washington University School of Medicine, Goldring completed his residency in internal medicine at the Peter Bent Brigham Hospital and he received his specialized rheumatology training at the Massachusetts General Hospital. His early research studies focused on the hormonal regulation of bone cells. He later investigated the vital relationship of osteoclasts to bone destruction.

Goldring has received multiple awards for his work in advancing the understanding of both rheumatoid arthritis and periprosthetic osteolysis, including the Carol Nachman Prize in Rheumatology, the Master's Award of the American College of Rheumatology, and the Paul Klemperer Award from the New York Academy of Medicine.

stimulated the macrophages or how it occurred, macrophages were not capable of destroying bone. Only osteoclasts have the capacity to do that.

Breakthroughs in science, as in life, often emerge when we take a detailed look at something we had, so far, failed to investigate. So it shouldn't have come as a surprise that we found crucial information in the detailed study of the soft fibrous tissue we'd all been striping away and discarding like debris.

Our work showed that when macrophages are stimulated by the ingestion of these particles, they, in turn, generate chemicals that are the products of their internal cellular activity, and it is these products that ultimately stimulate the osteoclasts (Figures 6.1 and 6.2).

We were the first to report such findings dealing with the molecular biology of this disease. It was now 1983. The macrophages generated two potent biochemical factors, two highly complex proteins: a cytokine called PGE_2 and an enzyme called *collagenase.* Cytokines are small proteins produced by one cell that can travel to another cell and influence the activity of that cell.

In those early days in 1983, knowledge about PGE_2 was incomplete because it had only recently been discovered. We now know that PGE_2 is a remarkable compound with a multiplicity of mind-bogglingly disparate functions throughout the body. For example, it protects the lining of the stomach from ulcers; aids in labor and the delivery of babies; helps regulate excretion of sodium through the kidney; and, unfortunately, facilitates the replication of the AIDS virus; *and* it stimulates osteoclasts. None of these functions were known at the time.

The function of the enzyme collagenase, on the other hand, was well known. It is the only enzyme in the body that can break down *collagen.* This was very instructive to our problem solving because collagen is the essential protein core of bone. Removing bone requires breaking down the collagen, which requires collagenase. The collagenase was also critical to our rodent experiments. If we simply placed this membrane on the skull of experimental mice, the membrane led to the resorption of the bone of the skull, just as in humans around the prostheses.

Subsequent research from many laboratories around the world on the molecular biology of this macrophage response established that, after ingesting these submicron particles, the macrophages produce a huge and complex cascade of proteins in addition to PGE_2 and collagenase, including many more enzymes and cytokines. It is the activity of the mosaic of these cellular products from the macrophages that ultimately stimulates the osteoclasts and causes the extraordinary bone destruction. Although explained here very briefly in a very simplified version, this research initiated the exemplary, detailed understanding of the amazingly complex molecular biology of the macrophage response to the particles.

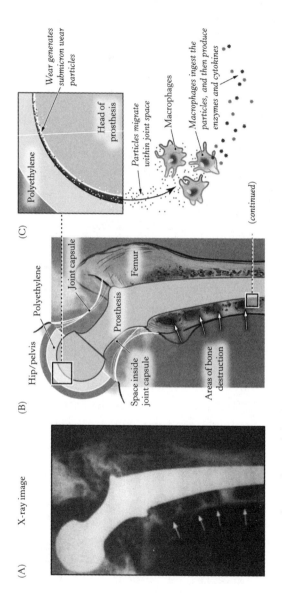

FIGURE 6.1 *The Biology of the Bone Destruction*

This figure illustrates the entire process of polyethylene wear leading to bone destruction. Figure 6.1A is the same x-ray shown in Figure 1.1 in Chapter 1, illustrating the bone destruction in the first case: that of Peter Dunn. Figure 6.1B is a drawing of that x-ray image, highlighting the bone destruction of the femur around the femoral prosthesis, and identifying the polyethylene and the hip capsule. Figure 6.1C enlarges a portion of the hip articulation to show the generation of the tiny wear particles of the polyethylene from motion in the joint. These particles escape and are subsequently ingested by macrophages. Then, the macrophages produce their proteins, called *cytokines* and *enzymes*. Printed with permission from Cassio Lynm, manager of Amino Creative, LLC, Stoneham, MA.

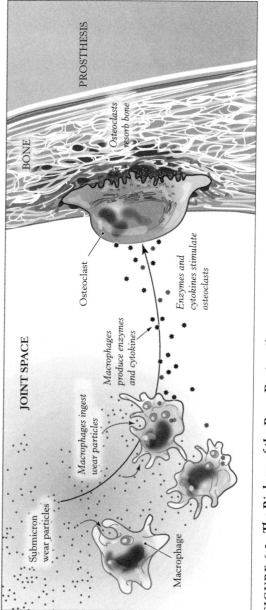

FIGURE 6.2 *The Biology of the Bone Destruction*

Figure 6.2 enlarges and completes the illustration shown in Figure 6.1C by presenting the ingestion of the particles by the macrophages and adding that the cytokines and enzymes stimulate a different cell type—the osteoclast—which in turn resorbs the bone. Printed with permission from Cassio Lynm, manager of Amino Creative, LLC, Stoneham, MA

This explanation was extremely important, even essential; but, alas, by itself, it was not enough. We still urgently needed to know how to *prevent* the bone destruction.

The artistry of the scientific advances in understanding the intricate and complex mechanism of this interaction of macrophages with the wear particles was thrilling to behold. At the same time, it pressured us to make another decision in the deep unknown. Two major options gave promise toward arresting this disease of bone destruction. With the first option, we could place our bets on pharmacologic solutions that a drug could be found that could block the biology involved—for example, disable the macrophages or interfere with the stimulation of the osteoclasts. Alternatively, we could gamble on reducing the wear. Both were totally uncertain, like "moon shots." Of the two, the approach to finding a drug appeared the more likely, particularly because the common nonsteroidal anti-inflammatory medicines such as Advil and so forth appeared to have a partial effect in blocking the actions of the macrophages in leading to bone destruction.

At this junction, now in the early 1990s, as occurred so often during the whole process, a key decision was made based purely on "feel," not on data. Conceptually, it was far more attractive to me to bet on stopping the fundamental cause—wear—than allowing wear to continue and then hope to block the effect of the wear. Either might work. Neither might work. But for style, not science, I favored trying our hand at decreasing wear.

Chapter 7

An Unexpected First Step

*Imagination should give wings to our thoughts ... and when
the moment comes to draw conclusions ... [it must be]
documented by the factual results of the experiment.*

—LOUIS PASTEUR

We had known from the very beginning that the hardest problem
to solve in a total hip implant was wear. All rubbing parts wear. In
automobile engines, the wear of the pistons is ameliorated by the
use of lubricating oil, a solution not possible in a human joint. In
normal human joints, wear is obviated by the marvelous, highly
complex, remarkable material called *articular cartilage*. Its unique
properties brilliantly reduce both friction and wear with biological mechanisms far too complex for us to reproduce artificially, at
least so far.

Skeptics of total hip replacements had always claimed that
wear in an artificial joint in humans was an insoluble problem
because of our inability to make cartilage or any other man-made
joint that would not wear badly inside the body under conditions
of human gait. Were they being proved right?

Replacing the human hip joint artificially is certainly a tough
problem. The inherent corrosive conditions inside the body are
hostile to virtually every foreign material. Most metals corrode.
Other materials degrade or oxidize. The body's active chemical,

and cellular and immune defenses attack or forcibly eject most others.

Add to these the severe mechanical demands of a hip. As noted before, many adults walk about two million steps per year. While simply walking around, the hip is loaded with more than twice the body weight. Vigorous activities raise the load across the hip joint to three to five times the body weight. For a 150-pound person, 300 to 750 pounds of load are driven through the hip joint. To bear that load consistently for 70 to 80 years is a massive challenge for any joint, biological or man-made. Nature handles it by covering the hip joint with this special tissue—cartilage—that is literally a marvel. One vastly simplified concept of how cartilage works is the idea that we actually "walk on water" every day. As the joint moves and is loaded, small amounts of the plain water (H_2O) trapped within the cartilage are squeezed slightly in and out of the cartilage with every step, and this water helps lubricate the joint.

Even to the present day scientists have not begun to comprehend how to mimic articular cartilage. They have, however, made engineering advances that allowed them to improve the design and function of certain types of total hip implants. Progressive developments of metal and ceramic materials were taking place as well, but polyethylene, which had initially shown great such promise, was still wearing.

As polyethylene wear increased, patients experienced other serious adverse effects even beyond the dire consequences of the bone destruction itself. Instead of continuing to rotate comfortably in the polyethylene socket, the ball of the hip joint (the *femoral head*) embedded itself progressively deeper and deeper into the plastic. Eventually, as that happened, the range of motion became severely reduced. With too much wear, the neck of the prosthesis began to impinge against the plastic and pry the artificial socket loose from the bone or, alternatively, this prying motion dislocated the hip altogether. At its most extreme, the ball wore through the plastic completely and the hip failed utterly.

All these complications, but particularly the bone destruction, generated a powerful, single focus on one problem: the *wear of the polyethylene.* This was unquestionably the dominating source of submicron particles.

By the end of the 1990s, a groundswell of dissatisfaction with polyethylene prompted a massive interest in so-called "alternate bearings" for total hip surgery. Metal-on-metal joints had been introduced long ago, about the same time as Charnley's polyethylene, but had gradually been outpaced by polyethylene joints, which worked better in most cases. Although ceramic-on-ceramic joints also had a long history with a small group of dedicated advocates, polyethylene vastly dominated the field. However, the belated recognition that polyethylene wear was deeply implicated in the widespread and devastating bone destruction initiated an intense race to find an alternative. Subsequent events would demonstrate disastrously that some of the risks involved in this pursuit of "any alternative bearing" were acutely misunderstood (see Chapter 15). Nevertheless, the race was on.

Because I had dedicated my life to the field of total hip surgery and had completed thousands of total hip operations, I had a deep commitment to addressing the enigma of finding a better articulation. Over the years, I'd developed respect as both a clinician and a research scientist. Working long hours, I divided my time between my patients and my research lab at the MGH. Considering this background and my access to some of the most accomplished medical scientists in the world as well, certain aspects of this desire were strong. Working against me, however, was the obvious limitation that neither I nor anyone connected with my lab was a materials scientist.

The arresting question was: Where to begin? Or even *how* to begin?

The track record of prior attempts to improve polyethylene was far from encouraging. *Dismal* may be a more accurate word. Three major efforts had been made previously to improve polyethylene, and one attempt to substitute another plastic (other than PTFE, of course) had been tried. All four of four were disastrous. Many patients had been badly harmed.

One company had added carbon fiber to the polyethylene, creating what was called *black poly*. Although adding constituents is a common tactic to improve the wear of plastics, this attempt was a substantial failure. Another company attempted to reduce the wear of the material by heating the surface under high pressure. This *heat-pressed polyethylene* was also a major failure. A third company introduced a product called *Hylamer,* marketed as "enhanced" polyethylene. However, it was prone to oxidation, which actually accelerated the wear and prompted early failure. An alternative approach, the substitution of a different class of plastics called *polycarbonates,* by yet another company was stunningly unsatisfactory and quickly withdrawn. In my view, for us to contribute to one more such disaster was unthinkable, and yet: What to do? Which of the three most likely avenues should we follow: metal on metal or ceramic on ceramic or try once again to improve polyethylene?

In medical school, we are taught to go immediately to the scientific literature, to garner the thoughts of everyone else who has ever been concerned with the problem, reaching all the way back to Aristotle, if you must. After you know what others have tried and after you have thought about what has been tried, we are then urged to look for a way to integrate that thinking with the current problem and take it further.

To me, this is a crippling approach. It inhibits free thought and bends your own thinking to the influence and limitations of everything that's gone before, when what you really need is to come up with something new!

It is far preferable to let your imagination run wild. The first step is really to "meditate" on the problem. Ignore the obstacles and allow your mind to run free. Stay open to innovative approaches. Move into a state of creative possibility and sustain it as long as you can. Practicality can wait.

This approach did, indeed, work for me at this critical juncture at the beginning of the 1990s, but in a most mysterious way. Thinking freely about our problem led me to an even more basic question: How would we know if we succeeded in inventing an innovative, new, wear-resistant plastic? What would tell us *before we began human experimentation* that we had, indeed, found a way that was likely to reduce wear enough to justify trying it in human beings? The thought was strange, but the solution was straightforward.

We urgently needed a way of testing wear that looked and functioned like the human hip in action. In other words, we needed *a hip simulator,* a complex research device that approximates closely what occurs inside the hip joint.

It was one of those moments where you want to cry, "Of course!"—a "lightbulb moment." But then reality kicked in. Various forms of hip simulators had existed since Charnley's experiments in the late 1950s, but none of them reflected fully and accurately the conditions in the human hip joint. Some simulators placed the joint upside down. Others did not control temperature. All were so unstable they required constant operator supervision.

To test potential hip replacement materials, we had to have a hip simulator that closely reflected the complexities of the human body when exposed to artificial materials in a moving joint over the equivalent of many, many years. If I wanted a hip simulator to do that, I'd have to build it myself. And that took me in an entirely different direction than I'd planned to go. Specifically, I'd have to *abandon* my goal of finding an innovative material for a new joint, at least for now. This was a huge and totally unexpected decision, but it was absolutely crucial.

The development of the hip simulator was a massive investment in many ways. Consuming ideas, personnel, and resources, it took three years to create our unique hip simulator. Our new design incorporated numerous features that we, as both clinicians and research scientists, knew to be vital, but had never been applied before (Figure 7.1). Five of the key innovations were the following:

1. **Load variation.** We built in the capacity to correlate the variations in weight, or load, across the hip joint in all phases of the human gait cycle—from the vastly lighter load of the swing phase of gait (while the foot is in the air) to the greater load during the weight-bearing phase of walking or even running. We also added the capacity to increase the load well beyond normal.

2. **Six degrees of freedom.** What engineers call "six degrees of freedom" means total freedom in every direction. Our hip simulator was capable of producing any and all motions a hip joint can make. Although this feature was underappreciated when we created it, it proved to be crucial (as discussed later). All hip simulators constructed before ours had sharply limited adaptability in the face of new information or different circumstances. It is far cheaper and faster to

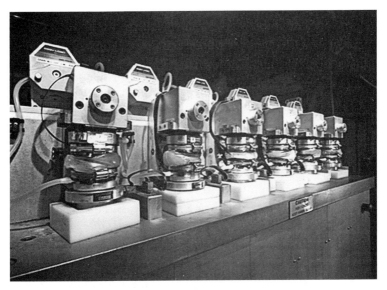

FIGURE 7.1 *The Hip Simulator*

Our new design for a hip simulator. Photo provided and reprinted with permission from Bruce Peterson, of Bruce Peterson Photography, 21 Wormwood St. Boston, MA. 02210.

ignore this flexibility. But, I felt we might encounter conditions that were previously unknown or ignored that I might need to explore (see Chapter 8).

3. **Upright position.** We put our hip in the upright position. Incomprehensibly, many hip simulators made the error of placing the hip upside down. This changes many of the conditions of human gait.

4. **Load cell.** In our desire to obtain the very most accurate information about the weight across the hip joint and to do it continuously, we attached a measuring device called a *load cell* to each artificial joint on the simulator to measure

continuously the weight crossing the hip joint. This had never been done before.

- **Twenty-four-hour automation.** Crucially, we needed this powerful machine to generate long-term data without an operator in attendance. To accomplish this, we made the strength, safety, and reliability of our hip simulator quite redundant. As a result, it could run safely day and night without anyone in attendance—a feature no other hip simulator had. Previous hip simulators could only run eight hours a day, with a technician in mandatory attendance. Running 24 hours a day *tripled* the output of our simulator.

When we had finally designed and created the simulator, we had to consider how long the testing should last. The FDA set the minimum testing requirement for new candidate materials for hip replacement articulations at five million cycles, or the equivalent of five million walking steps. Although that may seem like a large number, in fact it is not. Because, as mentioned, adults commonly walk two million steps a year, the FDA standard represented only about 2.5 years of walking—hardly a challenging test. Furthermore, we knew that bone destruction near the prosthesis often appeared only after 10 years or more. To improve on the existing polyethylene, any new materials would have to survive longer than the equivalent walking for that duration or even longer.

We set our own standard for testing at an unprecedented 29 to 30 million cycles, or the equivalent of 14.5 to 15 years of walking at two million steps per year. These severe requirements had never been used on any new potential material for a total joint.

We also introduced additional stringent criteria for testing. For example, we introduced tiny hard particles into the joint during testing because, in real life, small particles of metal or bone cement sometimes work their way into the joint.

When, at last, after three years the simulator was complete, we tested conventional polyethylene first. Because we knew the average wear rate was 100 microns per year for every two million steps, we required our hip simulator to demonstrate that wear to us. We were confident the results would confirm the full majesty of this comprehensive, complex, and sophisticated new machine.

After two million cycles, the polyethylene showed no wear at all. Not 98 microns. Not 50. None. How could that be? We checked again after four million cycles, then after seven million. No wear had occurred!

Our revolutionary new hip simulator had utterly failed!

Chapter 8

Flying Blind

Chance favors only the prepared mind.
—LOUIS PASTEUR

The most famous *failed* experiment in the history of science took place in 1887. During the late 19th century, physicists firmly believed that planets, light waves, and sound waves all moved through space in a hypothetical medium known as *ether.*

Albert Michelson was already renowned at the time for the creation of remarkable optical precision instruments. Just six years earlier, he had invented the *interferometer* to study the effect of Earth's motion on observed velocity. With Professor Edward Morley, he devised the ultimate experiment. Using the interferometer, they set out to measure the speed of Earth's movement through the ether. Their results changed science overnight.

The speed was *zero.*

If the experiment was accurate, it meant that ether simply didn't exist. Unable to believe it, the two scientists repeated the experiments many times over the next 42 years. The results were always the same.

Negative findings rarely get published. Nonetheless, the results of that first experiment were published in the *American Journal of Science.* A few years later, Albert Einstein developed the theory of special relativity, which marked the start of what is commonly called *the Second Scientific Revolution* and is still the most accurate model of motion at any speed.

Einstein had long suspected that Newton's mechanics and Maxwell's theories of electromagnetism were insufficient. In 1905, Einstein published his own alternative. It is keenly debated—but widely assumed—that the failure of Michelson and Morley to find evidence of ether was the final straw that propelled Einstein to hone his theory.

Curiously enough, the failed experiment also contributed to Michelson winning the Nobel Prize in Physics in 1907—a rare accolade for a "negative" result. Most experiments in science fail when the questions being asked are completely novel or the techniques are untested. However, it is uncommon for an experiment to fail when the techniques are basically well known and the questions being asked are modest. In fact, if the methods are largely established and the answer is known, that is not even research; it's just confirmation of existing information.

Our test of the hip simulator was, like the Michelson–Morley experiment, an attempt to confirm what was already taken for granted. We had built our hip simulator based on core assumptions. There was no reason to expect anything to go wrong. We were simply confirming what we knew: The old polyethylene wore under known conditions of human gait at a known rate of speed. Consequently, we were stunned there was no wear.

"We are clearly doing something wrong," I said. It was our practice to hold our weekly research meetings at night, because our days were filled with surgery, patient care, and experiments. That research meeting was dour, even somber. One of the guiding rules of my lab is that every person is "on" every project, regardless of whether they are assigned specifically to that project. Often I would survey the room silently while debating a failure or a perplexing issue, looking for eye contact with people who were not working explicitly on that issue, hoping to draw fresh thoughts or unanticipated contributions. That night I could not find any eye contact with anyone in the room. It was a major downer. It was then that I declared, "I don't know why there is no wear, but *when* we find out why—not *if* we find out why—we are going to know something about human gait that no one else in the world knows! And it will probably be very important."

So it began. Every facet of the experiment was challenged. We used faster and slower loading rates. We used heavier and lighter loads. We tried wider and narrower temperature ranges. We changed the characteristics of the synovial fluid. All to no avail.

"What if the pattern of motion we used was wrong?" I remarked with evident frustration to Danny O'Connor, the technician who ran the hip simulator. We had built in the back-and-forth pattern of hip motion, representing flexion and extension, based on the advice of the leading professor of tribology (wear) at the Massachusetts Institute of Technology (MIT) who had said "flexion–extension is 90% of the hip motion, particularly under load, and that is all you need."

"Flexion–extension may account for 90% of *observable* hip motion," I said. "But what is actually happening *inside* the hip? Does anyone know the specific pattern of motion *inside* the hip joint itself during one step or one gait cycle?"

No one knew because, amazingly enough, this question had never been asked before. As a result, it had never been studied. Everyone knew in great detail how the femur moved in relation to the pelvis. None of us had any idea what was happening *inside* the ball-and-socket joint.

Without knowing what was going on inside the hip, we couldn't identify what had gone wrong with our experiment and we couldn't answer a whole series of questions that had suddenly become quite relevant. When the hip was in motion, for example, would the movement of a single point on the front of the ball differ in length or direction from a point on the back of the ball? On reflection, it obviously had to. In fact, a point on the front of the ball *must* move in a very different pattern from a point on the back of the ball during many motions. For example, if you rotate your right hip so that the toes on your right foot point out to the right, a point on the front of the ball would move to the right, but a point on the back of the ball would move to the left.

After nearly 4000 years of medical observations, there was no information available on these questions. No one had thought to ask. Neither had we—until we set out to simulate the motion of a hip accurately.

To address the question, we had to rethink the pattern of motion we had built into the hip simulator.

"You're right," Danny said. "If flexion–extension were enough, the experiment would not have failed."

"Let's try incorporating the full motion of the femur," I proposed, realizing what a daunting task it would be. "We'll have to get all of the differing timing right. With every step, the pelvis tilts down and back up in very small increments. During the same time but not in unison, there is a slight internal and external rotation."

Looking at our hip simulator, Danny shook his head. "But to what degree?"

"We've got to get it precisely right," I noted. "Just the right amount of tilt and just the right amount of rotation, and also all motions must be correlated with the exact load pattern at just the right moment in the gait cycle."

"It's a good thing we built in six degrees of freedom!" Danny exclaimed.

We both laughed. The only hope we had of adding such complex motions into the gait pattern rested entirely on the capability for the six degrees of freedom we had built into the simulator from the beginning, simply on general principles, not knowing how crucial it would prove to be. This moment was our reward for making a good choice!

In the months to come, we faced many challenges. It proved to be much more difficult than we expected to identify the actual motion pattern produced by the femur on the surface of the ball during one gait cycle.

To find the answer, we ultimately needed to apply two very different, yet complementary, scientific methods: three-dimensional computer modeling and direct experimentation.

Our three-dimensional computer modeling was able to show us exactly what was happening inside the joint, but only to the degree that we fed it the correct data. To gather that data, we placed a short, sharp spike on the metal surface of the ball of the implant; went through one range of motion; and then analyzed the path this spike cut as it plowed through the surface of the polyethylene. The results of both of these studies reinforced each other and were a total surprise.

The basic back-and-forth motion of the hip is apparent. But, before the failure of the initial run of the simulator, the last thing we expected to discover was that, inside the hip joint itself, different points of the surface of the ball traced completely different courses altogether!

The internal patterns of motion were far more complex than was suggested by the apparent motion of the leg. Each point on the ball of the hip followed a path somewhat like a parallelogram, but its length and direction varied widely at different places on the ball (Figure 8.1).

Even more surprisingly, *each path overlapped the adjacent path,* a previously unknown crossing pattern. Fascinating! But what did it mean? To find out, we would now need to test the polyethylene again after we adjusted our simulator.

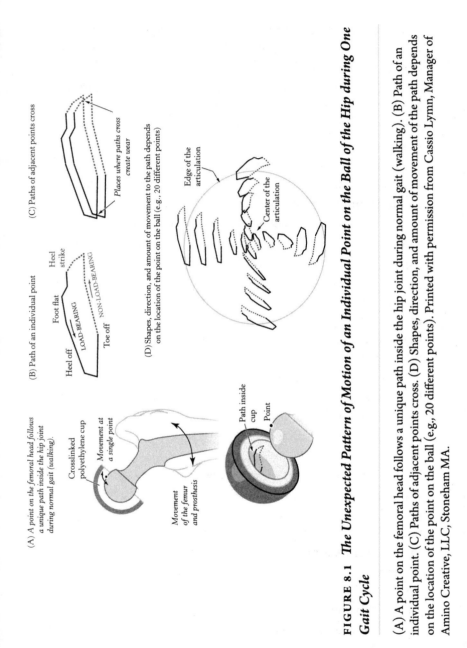

FIGURE 8.1 *The Unexpected Pattern of Motion of an Individual Point on the Ball of the Hip during One Gait Cycle*

(A) A point on the femoral head follows a unique path inside the hip joint during normal gait (walking). (B) Path of an individual point. (C) Paths of adjacent points cross. (D) Shapes, direction, and amount of movement of the path depends on the location of the point on the ball (e.g., 20 different points). Printed with permission from Cassio Lymn, Manager of Amino Creative, LLC, Stoneham MA.

We carefully incorporated the precise rotation and tilt into the motion pattern of the simulator, reproducing the overlapping parallelogram movements with the newly noted crossing pattern we had just discovered. We then reran the test.

Eureka! We had done it! The polyethylene wear in our simulator reproduced *exactly* the same rate of wear we had seen in patients. No prior hip simulator had ever been able to do this before, using these accurate human motion pathways. Correcting the motion pattern made all the difference. Moreover, this and subsequent extensive testing fully established that this previously unknown pattern of *overlapping* of the adjacent motion pathways to create a crossing pattern was absolutely fundamental to wear of the polyethylene. In fact, this critical observation immediately vitiated all the many prior publications of studies in polyethylene wear that *did not use the crossing pattern.*

My first reaction to the failure of the simulator had proved to be prescient. We had, indeed, learned something about gait that no one else in the world knew. And it had proved to be important. Even crucial.

Before we returned to our quest to find a new material for the hip replacement, we took the time to test another feature of polyethylene wear that had never been tested either: the effect of tiny, hard particles actually in the joint.

Occasionally, in real life a tiny flake of bone cement or a small shaving of metal from the implant would work its way into the joint of the hip replacement. We knew that these hard particles increased the wear. Having created an accurate hip simulator, we could now quantify that effect. We introduced several aggressive ways to challenge the wear, even adding hard particles slowly but continuously into the joint. And, indeed, all the hard particles made the wear much worse. So we now had one more stringent test to challenge any new material.

With the great success of these advances to our hip simulator, surgeons around the world began to rethink the effectiveness of the old simulators. We had raised the bar for testing by several magnitudes. Finding a way to ensure that the results in simulation mirrored the patients' experience exactly was a game changer. This new hip simulator design became the world standard. At last we had the capacity to test rigorously any new material we or anyone else might invent.

Now, three years later, in 1993, we were, again, squarely up against the fundamental question: Is it possible that we could invent a new material to reduce wear? We were determined to succeed, but where should we start?

The first option, metal-on-metal hip replacements was a real possibility. The metal-on-metal total hips were known to generate, by far, the largest number of particles, and those particles were really minute—in nano-size dimensions. But, despite the theoretical problems this huge number of particles implied, the track record for these implants was excellent. Large numbers of patients had been well served by them over many years. In fact, I am a coauthor of a report of a successful metal-on-metal total hip replacement prostheses retrieved after 25 years of excellent service. Still, I had long worried about metal on metal as a long-term solution—especially without the benefit of lubrication. Perhaps if I went in that direction, I might come up with some new form of lubrication.

Alternatively, over the years, many patients had also done very well with the next possible choice: ceramic-on-ceramic joints. Ceramic material is considered more biocompatible than metal. Yet, the failure of several of the early ceramic-on-ceramic designs from chipping or fractures of either the ceramic ball or the ceramic socket left me with some concerns. Nevertheless, a deeper investigation into these failings might be fruitful.

Our third option, metal on polyethylene, had some special values to me because this combination was considered "more forgiving." This phrase reflects that, even if the surgical technique was slightly less than perfect, these implants would survive. Metal-on-metal and ceramic-on-ceramic devices are far less forgiving. The surgical technique for these two is more exacting, and, in any case in which the hip dislocated, the metal ball coming out of the joint caused far less damage as it slid across the soft polyethylene than if it scraped against a metal or ceramic socket.

If we elected to turn our focus on polyethylene, it would mean launching into the wild unknown. To improve polyethylene ourselves—a challenging prospect, because all three previous attempts by the three largest device manufacturers in the United States had unequivocally failed—was daunting, to say the least.

We were faced with the decision of risking all our talents and resources on one of these three types of devices, without any way of knowing which path might prove successful. It was an all-or-nothing gamble. The entire enterprise teetered on the brink of folly anyway, because no one in our lab was a materials engineer or a polymer specialist in the first place!

We were flying blind.

Many successful research decisions are based on a new concept. Others are based on a new technique or a fresh application. Some are serendipitous. A few are pure luck. With 20/20 hindsight, 25 years later, I can say the success of my choice was a result of serendipity.

After carefully assessing the pros and cons of solving the problem of bone destruction by improving metal joints, ceramic joints, or metal-on-polyethylene joints, I chose the third type, hoping to modify the polyethylene to decrease wear.

To this day, I can't quite say why. No doubt it was a largely subconscious decision, yet it felt strangely comfortable. Maybe it was because I had extensive previous experience with both metal on metal and metal on polyethylene, and I "liked" the metal-on-polyethylene joints better. In the end, it was one of the most momentous decisions of my life, and it was made, like many difficult decisions, in the absence of adequate information.

Having made that decision brought me back to the nagging question I had from the start: What was causing the bizarre, unexplained, and unique type of polyethylene wear that generated those vast numbers of submicron particles with every step?

It was here that serendipity came to the rescue. It emerged from our decades-long projects we had been pursuing for other reasons, reasons that had absolutely nothing to do with bone destruction or polyethylene wear rates.

Incidentally, Charnley's huge contributions also provided major serendipitous help—in fact, twice. After the disappointing failure of PTFE, Charnley dedicated his laboratory to a search for a better plastic material. Luckily, a local salesman of plastic piping heard that "some crazy Englishman was putting plastics in the human body."

"Why not try my plastic?" the salesman asked, when he showed up unannounced at Charnley's door. "We use *ultrahigh-molecular weight polyethylene* in everything from soil pipes to sewage pipes in hotels. If it can transport urine and feces, it must be OK to use in the body, right?"

Charnley, after hearing this bizarre pitch, threw him out; but, his head technician ran after the guy in the parking lot. "Give me a little of this stuff," the technician said. "I'll try it at night when the boss isn't here. If it works, you'll hear from me; if not, ..."

It worked, and spectacularly well. For the next 40 years, that specific form of polyethylene was the first-choice material for total hip replacements throughout the world.

Charnley's other moment of serendipity occurred when he was just starting out. As he explored the possibility of creating artificial hips, one of his earliest challenges was to figure out how to get the metal thigh piece to stick to the femur. It occurred to him that dentists fix artificial teeth somehow in people's mouth all the time. So he went to the dental school in Manchester, United Kingdom, and spoke to Dennis Smith, the materials scientist who selected the dental materials.

"What kind of plastic do you use in the body?" Charnley asked him.

"Methyl methacrylate," was the answer.

Smith hadn't really understood the question and gave Charnley the wrong answer. But it worked! Charnley had meant really *inside the body* and Smith replied to the question as if Charnley meant inside the mouth. "Inside the mouth" and "inside the body" are entirely different. But the wrong answer worked. Forever after, Charnley used methyl methacrylate, which is the chemical name of the plastic commonly called *bone cement*, to anchor the artificial parts of the prosthesis to the bone. In fact, during the early days of total hip surgery, the methyl methacrylate he used had the same pleasant pink color of healthy gums, because the acrylic dental cement had originally been designed for use in the mouth. Ironically, when Charnley received the Lasker Award (Figure 2.3), the committee specifically cited his "introduction of the use of methyl methacrylate as a bone cement."

Our serendipity story is this. As part of my laboratory's mission to improve total hip surgery, I had developed an active program for analysis of those total hip implants that had been recovered after use in patients. Many were obtained from operating rooms during revision surgeries. Even more valuable, however, were those special implants that had *not* failed. As tactfully as possible, we invited a carefully selected, small group of patients to donate their hips back to us when they "no longer needed them"—that is to say, after they passed away. Recognizing the value of this research, many patients were glad to help.

These autopsy specimens provided us with information that was simply not available from the "reoperation specimens" that had been removed after the failure of the total hip operation. One massively important difference was that we were able to obtain and to study all the surrounding bone as well. Autopsy specimens were also free from secondary changes related to the failure of the implants, such as loosening, which caused additional damage after the implant was no longer fixed to the skeleton. For us, serendipity came from reexamining these retrieved specimens, all of which were available only because we had collected them for entirely different purposes. But this time we were looking for the answer to the puzzle of why tiny particles wore off. We studied 148 used polyethylene implants with a sophisticated electron microscope technique called *scanning electron microscopy* (SEM).

These findings were pivotal. And they simultaneously validated once more the brilliant observation of one of the most productive scientists the world has ever known: Louis Pasteur. His work resulted in crucial applications and theories that laid the foundation of many branches of science, including the germ theory of disease, the development of numerous vaccines, the establishment of the principles of pasteurization, and also the advancement of knowledge of the structure of organic compounds.

In a speech in 1854 he said, "*dans les champs de l'observation, le hasard ne favorise que les esprits préparés*" ("in the field of observations, chance favors only the prepared mind"). This had been one of the mottoes of my laboratory from the very start.

The SEM studies led us to a chance observation—one that was simultaneously seductive and fragile. It was hard to ignore the fact that this observation would have had zero impact on us if we had not been searching for the mechanism of wear of polyethylene. That search was our "prepared mind." The key observation from the SEM studies was that certain molecules of the polyethylene had changed their orientation.

At the molecular level, the individual strands of polyethylene molecules ordinarily have a helter-skelter orientation, like spaghetti in a bowl. We discovered that, in a very specific region of the polyethylene—just below the worn areas—after they had been in human use, the strands were no longer helter-skelter. They were all lined up parallel to each other, aligned in one direction. In the body, after being exposed to repeated flexion and extension in the joint, they had aligned with the direction of movement.

This was a "chance observation" for many reasons. The change in orientation was limited to a small area, an area that could have been easily overlooked. It was a chance observation also because, even if the reorientation had been seen but we were we not looking for a reason for the unusual mechanism of the origin of the tiny particles of wear, the observation would have no reason to appear to be important and would likely have been ignored.

But, in our quest to understand the wear of the polyethylene, this realignment was so distinctive that it made us curious. This thin reed of an observation suggested a concept so fresh, so new, and so tentative, we couldn't help but wonder: *Could this realignment be the crucial element in creating the unusual form of wear that underlies the bone destruction?*

To test this possibility, we would need to prevent this realignment. But how? If we did find a way to interrupt that reorientation, we would be able to establish whether it was related to the unique form of wear. It was always possible, however, that we might encounter adverse effects from preventing the reorientation as well. But, could this chance discovery actually be the solution to bone destruction? I thought it might.

Excited by this grand but unproved hypothesis, we forged ahead.

Chapter 9

The Gamble Pays Off

The important thing is to never stop questioning.
—ALBERT EINSTEIN

The agony and the ecstasy of total hip replacement was epitomized perfectly by Patrick Sands. A tall, blond athlete with a buoyant personality, he enjoyed a thriving business as a tennis pro in Florida.

A younger Patrick had played the professional tennis circuit at a very high level, but over time, he had gradually developed a stiffness in his hips that impaired his game. He couldn't follow through on the strokes as he had before. And when he tried to move through the pain, his form suffered.

After a few years, he managed to find a coach who helped him adjust his swing to compensate, but by then, the pain was getting worse. X-rays revealed he had congenital underdevelopment of the hip socket. It was unusual in a man, because 95% of people with this condition are female.

"Your hip socket is more shallow than it should be," his doctor told him. "For some reason, it did not develop deeply enough." He pointed to the x-ray. "A normal socket would extend much deeper than this."

Patrick frowned at the x-ray. He had to admit the hip socket did not look quite right, even to his untrained eyes. "But I can walk," he said. "And I've been playing tennis all these years!"

"Yes," the doctor nodded. "That's been because you've been compensating successfully. It's actually quite amazing. The mechanics of the joint are really compromised."

"Why has it just started hurting now?"

"Over time, the joint wears out," the doctor explained. "You've probably felt an ache in your joints for a long time, but lately, it's become impossible to ignore, am I right?"

Patrick shrugged. "I thought it was just soreness."

"It's arthritis. In both hips. And it's not going to get any better."

"What can you give me for it?"

"A referral. You need to see an orthopaedic surgeon."

By the time I saw Patrick in 1979, his symptoms had become quite severe. It was necessary to carry out total hip replacements on both hips, and at that time they were both cemented total hips.

This was during the awkward period when bone destruction had been identified as *cement disease*, but no cementless devices had been developed. I explained the situation to Patrick, letting him know the risks. I said that his hip replacements would likely last 10 years or so, but beyond that, we were uncertain. Despite the potential time limit, the procedure would restore much of his mobility and eliminate the chronic pain in both hips that was starting to keep him awake at night. I was glad to let him know, too, that we were actively researching the problem and hoped to see new developments in the coming years.

The surgery went well and Patrick's recovery was straightforward. After he healed fully from surgery itself, he was amazed by the absence of pain. Over the years, pain had become a perpetual presence, increasingly inhibiting his movement. With the pain and stiffness gone, he felt like a new man.

"Can I go back to playing tennis again?" Patrick asked eagerly.

"Let's be cautious about activities that pound the hip," I advised him. "Golf is fine. With tennis, I'd recommended doubles, rather than singles. Even then, be ready to call out 'Yours!' to your partner at strategic times. Teaching tennis is OK, as long as you do it from the sidelines."

Patrick's eyes glazed over, masking his disappointment. I could see his heart had been set on going back to *playing* tennis, but he followed my instructions faithfully, at first.

His recovery was excellent. Within a few months, he returned to the very busy life of a popular tennis pro. Every time I saw him, he was doing better than ever. It was a delight to see his rapid return to health.

In my clinical office, I often have the privilege of seeing one happy postoperative patient after another. It is one of the real pleasures of my work as a surgeon, to put an end to the deep, daily grief that patients often suffered, by giving them total hip replacements. Their joy and gratitude afterward were some of my greatest rewards. However, those with bone destruction were my worst nightmares.

Patrick was one of the most jubilant. "I feel like I could play again," he would tell me with a mischievous twinkle in his eye.

One day, in between lessons, a fellow tennis pro lobbed a ball at him across the net. Patrick hit it back. They struck up a lively set that left him elated. Before he knew it, Patrick was back in the game. He experienced no pain or stiffness. For the first time in more than a decade, he could follow through the hips on his swings. It gave his returns a new power.

The temptation to return to competition was overwhelming. Tentatively, he found a partner and signed up for men's doubles and invited his former coach to sit in the stands and watch. The coach was excited by what he saw. "I think you've got what it takes," he said. "If we start training now, I'll bet we can get you to the state finals!"

Two years later, Patrick won the state championship for men's doubles in his age group. An impressive feat, because the state of Florida represents a very high level of excellence in tennis. Patrick was in ecstasy. The agony came eight months later when he dove to return a serve and a searing pain shot through his hips. The second time it happened, it left him crumpled on the ground. He was frantic.

"Everything was going great!" he moaned, limping into my office one day. "What happened?"

My examination revealed that his right thigh implant had come loose. The x-ray showed extensive bone destruction in the right femur and moderately extensive destruction on the left side as well. The tragic reality was that the most dynamic, active implant patients suffered the most rapid damage to their new artificial joints. Regrettably, the only solution was reoperation. Patrick's case and others like his drove me even more to exert every possible effort to solve the problem of bone destruction around total hip prostheses.

Once I decided to risk everything on the gamble that we could somehow alter polyethylene to decrease wear significantly, and based specifically on our nascent, fledgling hypothesis, I knew I was going to need to enlist experts in biomedical engineering and polymer science.

As luck would have it, I already had one of the top experts from MIT working with me in another capacity, supervising one of his PhD candidates working in my laboratory on bone cement. Ed Merrill was a professor of chemical engineering at MIT. He was also my neighbor in Belmont, Massachusetts. We'd been friends since the early 1970s, when we worked together on a massive grant application—a program–project grant for the National Institutes of Health (Profile 9.1).

One day in the lab, I approached him and said, "We have just discovered that hip implants create a curious reorientation of the long, intertwining molecules in polyethylene. Can you prevent this from happening?"

"Of course!" Ed replied happily.

When I asked him just how he proposed to do that, he replied prophetically, "We'll just crosslink the polymer with electron beam irradiation."

As it turned out, the term "just" covered a multiplicity of problems and created an abundance of anxiety. The concept was that exposure of the polyethylene to the high-energy beams of electron radiation was capable of linking one strand of polymer to the next, in a process called *crosslinking*. Using this electron beam (e-beam) irradiation to create the crosslinking, the movement of individual strands was dramatically reduced. This process had the potential to bind the strands in their original helter-skelter pattern and keep them from lining up in the reoriented pattern that I believed was creating the unusual wear in such small particles, which ultimately led to the bone destruction. It would mean creating an entirely new material for use in total hip replacements (e-beam crosslinked polyethylene), then testing it to assess its advantages in our new hip simulator. If that worked, two things would follow. First, it would support our hypothesis. Second, it might lead to a low-wear polyethylene suitable for testing in people.

Crosslinked polyethylenes of other types generated by different means were already being used in industry to improve resilience against wear, temperature changes, mechanical strength, and other properties. The interconnection of molecules by a network of crosslinking bonds made these polymers extremely stable and resistant to wear. If the same process worked on our

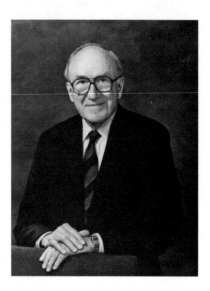

Image courtesy of and reprinted with permission from
Professor Ed Merrill.

Following a proven pathway from Boston's Roxbury Latin
High School to Harvard, Ed Merrill became entranced
there by chemical engineering. This fascination for chemical engineering not only led him to graduate from Harvard
in just three years, but also to complete his DSc at the
Massachusetts Institute of Technology (MIT) in chemical
engineering, similarly, in just three years.

After a brief stint in industry, Ed returned to MIT to teach
and do research. But consider the fact that, at that time (in
1950), MIT offered but one single course in polymers. As

the field expanded dramatically thereafter, Ed cotaught a polymer course with Paul Flory, who in 1974 became the first and only Nobel laureate ever to be awarded this special prize for work on polymers. Over many years, Ed's research projects on polymers often involved the use of the electron beam generator at MIT, a powerful source of energy that could produce chemical bonds between two independent strands of a given polymer.

His wide-ranging research interest in polymers led naturally to many studies of the issues of how human blood flows within plastic (polymer) tubing, such as in crucial medical devices as diverse as renal dialysis machines and heart–lung pumps. His extensive background in the applications of polymers to medical problems generated a very natural association with our team in our efforts to make a wear-resistant polyethylene.

Worldwide recognition has come to Ed in many forms. He is unusual, if not unique, in being a member of all four of the most prestigious national organizations reflecting his scientific and engineering career—namely, the American Academy of Arts and Sciences, the American Institute of Medical and Biological Engineering, the Institute of Medicine of the National Academies, and the National Academy of Engineering. He holds 70 patents and has published 250 refereed scientific articles as well as one textbook (which becomes very important later).

new polyethylene in hip replacement devices, we might just have a solution!

With this promising possibility in mind, we hired a dynamic young polymer scientist, Orhun Muratoglu (Profile 9.2), who had just completed his PhD at MIT in polymer science, and got to work. Our project had now become a joint venture between the MGH and MIT. I had no doubt we now had the intellectual horsepower we needed in polymer science to drive the investigation forward.

When we began our crosslinking program in 1993, the biomedical applications of crosslinking polymers were only beginning to be explored; but, strangely enough, the process itself had been around since prehistoric times. Around 1600 BC, the first major civilization in Mexico, the Olmec, learned that if they mixed the sap from white morning glory vines with the latex extracted from rubber trees, it transformed the latex into something very elastic.

Although the Olmecs had no idea that organic compounds in the sap were creating strong crosslinks in the polymer, they did make use of this newly elastic rubber to create a vitally important object: a bouncing ball. The invention of the rubber ball gave rise to a ball game that would become one of the central rituals for all ancient Mesoamerican cultures for centuries. The Aztec word *Olmec* literally means "rubber people"—an apt name, as they were the first to crosslink a polymer.

At MIT we applied the e-beam irradiation to crosslink the polyethylene in the hopes of increasing its resistance against wear. Although both Ed and Orhun were confident that crosslinking would successfully alter the polymer, our first hurdle was to determine how *much* radiation and how *fast* the energy from the e-beam should be applied. Because no one had specifically crosslinked this polyethylene in this way before, and because it

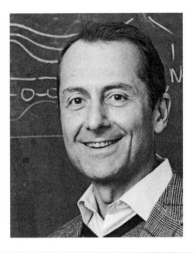

Image courtesy of and reprinted with permission from
Professor Orhun Muratoglu.

Orhun Muratoglu was born in the small town of Erzurum
in eastern Turkey, in the mountainous region near Iran
and the former Soviet Republic. Although the small town
was deeply conservative, he benefited from growing up in
a progressive family. Not knowing that his departure from
Erzurum would lead him to Boston, he insisted on going
to a boarding school in Istanbul when he was 11 years old.
He succeeded in convincing his parents to part with their
firstborn, and Orhun landed himself in Galatasaray Lisesi,
a French/Turkish high school in the heart of the bustling
metropolis of Istanbul.

   He studied at the Lisesi until he started college at
Bosporus University, where he decided that industrial
engineering would be a good career choice. However,
within two years, he realized his heart was set on study-
ing and understanding how materials worked. During that

interval, he met his future wife, Tonya, and together they departed for the United States. Tonya enrolled at Vassar and Orhun began the program in materials science at nearby Rensselaer Polytechnic Institute.

After receiving his bachelor of science degree in materials science from Rensselaer, where he received the Matthew Albert Hunter Prize for Outstanding Academic Achievement, Orhun was selected to join the rigorous PhD Program in Polymer Science and Technology at MIT, funded by a DuPont fellowship.

Orhun honed his problem-solving skills at MIT, where he prepared himself for the upcoming long journey in becoming, first, a team member, and then a leader at the Harris Orthopaedic Laboratory at the MGH. There he developed multiple innovative ways of modifying and altering the chemical structure of ultrahigh-molecular weight polyethylene, the unique polymer used worldwide in total joint implants. He created several novel forms of that material that are vastly more suitable for long-term use in not only more sedentary elderly patients, but also in more active, young candidates for total joint surgery.

His work has been recognized by his promotion to the rank of professor of orthopaedic surgery at Harvard Medical School and the positions of Alan Gerry scholar, codirector and then director of the Harris Orthopaedic Laboratory, and director of the Technology Implementation Research Center at the MGH. He received the HAP Paul Award, given by the International Society for Technology in Arthroplasty, three times and the prestigious Marshall R. Urist Young Investigator Award from the American Academy of Orthopaedic Surgeons. Orhun has published more than 80 refereed scientific articles and holds more than 70 national and international patents.

was a particularly complex plastic, finding the right amounts of radiation was going to take a little experimentation. We expected it to be a perfunctory matter of adjusting the dosages. It proved to be far more frightening than we anticipated.

In early tests, the energy from the e-beam radiation actually "melted" the polyethylene. With most substances, "melting" transforms a solid into liquid, as when ice melts. But polyethylene is strangely different. When it melts, it actually expands slightly, keeping its same basic shape, and transforms from an opaque white solid to become quite translucent. This polyethylene has one other unusual characteristic called *shape memory*. If you cool it after it "melts," it remembers the shape it had before melting and it returns precisely to that former shape.

Melting. That was odd. But what was worse, was that some of the specimens burst into flames! Even more alarming were the explosions.

My lab is in a remote part of the MGH, far from the areas of my patient care and surgery, although some of the personnel engaged in research and patient care overlap. The e-beam radiation experiments were done even farther away, at MIT. The explosions were the one event in 50 years that prompted instantaneous transfer of information from the experiment to me in my clinical office, temporarily interrupting the care of a patient. Because of the inherent precautions we always used during e-beam irradiation, no one was injured physically, but the psychic damage was real.

The translucency wasn't so bad, but it was hard to imagine that any potential manufacturer, let alone any patient, would be interested in hips that could potentially explode or burst into flames during manufacture. With our "new and improved" but highly combustible polymer, we were at a full stop.

After massive consternation and extensive research, we finally identified the problem. When the issue was fully revealed, the explanation proved to be an already-known phenomenon, one that had not yet been seen in this polyethylene under these circumstances. It had a wonderful name: *adiabatic heating*. Adiabatic heating occurs when the addition of energy or heat to a chemical reaction actually speeds up the chemical reaction until *the reaction itself* generates even more heat.

When we began to crosslink the polyethylene, the e-beam irradiation added heat. Then, the chemical process of crosslinking generated extra heat—enough extra heat that the polymer either melted or burst into flames. Or exploded.

Now that we knew that, we could anticipate additional heat from the crosslinking itself, and we knew we had to reduce the radiation accordingly. This sounds easier than it was, because the heat did not build up at a steady rate. So, we needed to calibrate the radiation to account for the heat generated from the crosslinking, slowing the radiation down progressively as the crosslinking reaction gained speed.

By further extensive experimentation, we succeeded. With the problems caused by adiabatic heating solved, we could consistently generate crosslinked polyethylene without incident. But this would not be our last problem of heat transfer during crosslinking

I was reminded that Isaac Newton said, "If I have ever made any valuable discoveries, it has been owing more to patient attention, than to any other talent."

By 1995, I had been heavily committed to the quest for a new material for a long five years. And my pursuit of the nature of the bone destruction problem now covered two decades, starting with the sheets of macrophages in Peter Dunn's biopsy in 1974. The powerful insights that particle disease was caused by both bone cement particles and polyethylene wear particles were invaluable, but they were only steps along the way to solving the initial problem. Once I had committed to trying to find a better articulation for a total hip, I'd been forced to stop for three years to invent and perfect the new hip simulator so I could study the wear. Then we had to come up with an innovative polymer to test.

Newton was right about the need for patience. All of this had taken a lot more time than I would ever have anticipated, but my gamble had paid off. E-beam crosslinking had given us a completely new type of polyethylene for biomedical use.

For the first time, we could really begin to test our theory. We had the two essential ingredients: a precisely representative hip simulator and a new material that held the exciting promise of a far greater resistance against wear.

It was time to bite the bullet and test our crosslinked polyethylene.

Chapter 10

Success at Last!

*It has to do with curiosity. It has to do with people wondering
what makes something do something. And then to discover, if
you try to get answers, that they are related to each other . . . .
What we're looking for is how everything works—what makes
everything work.*

—RICHARD FEYNMAN

This was the pivotal moment. By 1995, after five years of preparation, we finally had a new, promising, but untested, material to examine plus a sophisticated means to test it.

Legions of patients had proved that conventional polyethylene wore at about an average of 100 microns per year, about the thickness of a human hair. When the earlier test of conventional polyethylene on our first design of the simulator showed no wear, we knew the hip simulator was wrong and did not represent a valid test. We put the intervening years to good use by creating an accurate hip simulator, calibrated specifically to the complex human gait pattern. Then, upon retesting the conventional polyethylene, the redefined simulator had reproduced precisely what actually happens to conventional polyethylene in life in patients. So now, with great anticipation and some measure of anxiety, we were ready to assess our new candidate material to the same exacting standards.

We tested the crosslinked polyethylene for seven million walking cycles. "No wear" had been bad news before, when we knew there should have been wear. Now, for the refined simulator testing of our crosslinked material, *the result was exactly the same: no wear.* But this time, zero wear was a joyful result!

Our surprise and delight were hard to contain. We had been hoping that, if successful, we could reduce wear, not eliminate it. If our new material had significantly reduced wear, we would have been pleased. The actual outcome went far beyond that. We had exceeded our expectations. The hypotheses appeared to work. Suddenly, *crosslinked polyethylene looked very promising.*

But, was this the acid test? Not at all. The inadequacy of that result lay in the fact that the FDA requirement of five million test cycles for any candidate material for the articulation for a total hip replacement—although it had been the country's standard for 25 years—represented only about 2.5 years of adult walking, as mentioned earlier. This duration was nowhere near the life expectancy of the average patient receiving a total hip replacement and was far less than that of a young, vigorous patient. What would happen after 25 or 30 million cycles (12.5–15 years of walking)? And so, back to more testing.

We were also vividly aware that we had tested our material under one ideal set of circumstances and, in life, circumstances are rarely ideal. I wouldn't be satisfied the material would meet our needs until it had survived more extreme conditions. How would crosslinked polyethylene stand up to our more severe testing and against small pieces of metal or bone cement in the joint? What if extreme motions in the joint banged the femoral component against the edge of the crosslinked polyethylene?

Working the simulator around the clock, we tested each of these conditions systematically, starting with our own self-imposed requirement to assess wear after 29 or 30 million cycles, not five million. Here, the results were really "unbelievable." Again, no wear! There was no wear after subjecting the crosslinked polyethylene to very prolonged testing on the hip simulator that approximated 14.5 years of walking. This result was a striking reduction in wear—a complete absence. This remarkable decrease in wear implied that, if similar reduction occurred in patients, we might sharply curtail or even cure this bone destruction.

No test of this duration had ever been carried out in the past. The basic reason was that it would simply take too long to test 15 years of walking at the average pace in any existing hip simulator before ours. Naturally, any simulation would have to be run at or near actual walking speeds. A faster pace would not test actual conditions.

As mentioned earlier, specifically because we had anticipated just this problem, we deliberately created our hip simulator with the capacity to run 24 hours a day without supervision. As mentioned previously, all the other simulators could only run eight hours a day under the supervision of a technician. At that rate, to complete 29 million cycles, such prolonged testing would take more than 1.5 years—*for just one test!* Even running simulations 24 hours a day, it took us *six months* to run each test. Nevertheless, in our view, such testing was essential. We ran 29 million cycles in our lab and, for confirmation, an outside lab ran 30 million cycles on a duplicate of our machine.

Both tests showed no detectable wear. It was a genuine triumph.

Moreover, we found that, although the small hard pieces of metal, cement, or ceramic did increase the wear of our crosslinked polyethylene, the wear produced was vastly less than in conventional polyethylene. And, if the thigh piece did bang into the edge of the crosslinked polyethylene at the extreme of motion, the damage to the spot where it hit was dramatically less than with the old polyethylene.

This remarkable moment was the dramatic realization of our fondest hopes—the confirmation of our fragile hypotheses. At least in the laboratory setting, we'd found the solution we'd been searching for all these years.

Thrilled as we were to have found a possible way to save millions of future total hip patients from failure, pain, fractures, and reoperations, there was much to do. Like all scientists, we were professional skeptics. It is hardwired.

"Well, there must be *some* wear, however undetectable," Orhun remarked, when he saw the results, "although it's still a massive reduction in wear compared with conventional polyethylene."

"You must be right," I replied. "Because otherwise, we would have defied the laws of physics and invented a *perpetual motion machine!*" But because we did not, even the wear that must be occurring was so very minimal that the outlook was favorable.

But immediately, we had to address another materials problem: oxidation.

After so many successes, we never expected all our research to end up in a fish tank. But that's what happened next.

I realized there were remained two niggling issues in the back of my mind. Crosslinked polyethylene had one single property that made it less resistant to fatigue than conventional polyethylene. This was because, as the e-beam radiation reduced wear, it weakened the fatigue resistance slightly. Second, the radiation left behind *free radicals*—very active chemical agents that promote a form of deterioration called *oxidation*.

My question then was: How important are these two problems for our crosslinked polyethylene? Before we moved on, I had to be sure we'd addressed these issues.

We turned our attention first to free radicals. With our world-class polymer scientists on the job, they soon discovered we could eliminate nearly all free radicals by—strangely enough—melting the polyethylene after the e-beam radiation. This was good, and it got rid of the free radicals, but the melting itself also slightly reduced fatigue resistance further. Although it was unlikely that the total amount of reduction would cause problems in human use, there was no way to know for sure. We would have no way of finding out for certain until our promising new material was put to the test in patients. This was a risk we and our patients would have to take.

Next, we needed a test for oxidation. That's where the fish tank came in.

In the midst of our state-of-the-art medical research laboratory at one of the finest hospitals in the world, we, three highly specialized scientists, dunked our cutting-edge crosslinked polyethylene components into an ordinary fish tank from the hobby store! We bubbled oxygen through water at body temperature in the fish tank containing crosslinked polyethylene samples. This simple—and ridiculously inexpensive—test proved to be the best test for oxidation. The only serious limitation was that the test couldn't be accelerated. Oxygen bubbled up slowly through the body-temperature water in real time, so these tests also took real time. But, after our crosslinked polyethylene had eventually spent years in the fish tank, we were quite relieved to find that it showed no signs of deterioration from oxidation.

As we moved toward the threshold of the use of this remarkable material in patients, my imagination took hold once more.

The fact that crosslinked polyethylene showed no wear at all was so astonishing that it gave me a radical new idea. The resulting development was totally unexpected and proved to be remarkably valuable.

The average diameter of the ball at the top of the femur that fits snugly into the hip socket is roughly 1.5 inches in women and two inches in men. Yet, the femoral balls in every one of Charnley's polyethylene total hip replacements were only less than one inch, because he found that bigger heads generated more wear.

This situation was suddenly intriguing, considering the fact that we had just created a new material that, in the simulator, showed no wear. "No wear" proved to be true regardless if we tested a femoral ball of less than one inch in diameter (22 millimeters) or one of slightly more than one inch (32 millimeters)— the largest diameter of ball used for metal-on-plastic total hips from 1957 onward. What if the wear resistance of this material was so great that even a normal-size femoral head could be used?

That would be fantastic! It would represent a huge advance in total hip surgery.

Understanding the vast importance and great appeal of a larger ball takes us back to the first total hip replacement that Charnley designed, probably around 1955. In his very original design, Charnley used a femoral ball with a diameter of 41.5 millimeters (Figure 10.1). But, the PTFE wore so rapidly he was forced to use smaller and smaller heads. He finally settled on a ball size of less than one inch (22 millimeters). That size allowed him to build in a thicker layer of PTFE to provide additional durability despite the wear.

Even when he first introduced conventional polyethylene in 1962, Charnley adhered to the same principle. His arguments and his experiences about using small balls were so persuasive that, even four decades later, many of the total hip

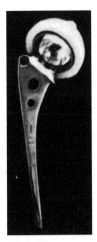

FIGURE 10.1 *Charnley's Original Total Hip Design*

Although Charnley is widely known for his advocacy of a very small femoral ball diameter (22.5 millimeters), he was driven to the small head size because of the wear of the plastic. Before he encountered this rapid wear of the plastic, he wished to use a large head, as shown here (41.5-millimeter femoral ball diameter) in his original design of a total hip. The dramatic reduction of wear caused by crosslinking eliminated the need for a small head. With crosslinked polyethylene, the use of larger heads has two strong advantages: increasing the range of motion and reducing sharply the risk of dislocation.

Published with permission from BMJ Publishing Group, LTD, from Surgery of the Hip-Joint: Present and Future Developments. Charnley J. From *Br Med J*. 1960 Mar 19:1(826) Figure 8B.

replacements around the world were still being made with 22-millimeter-diameter femoral heads. The largest ball that anyone used in those days was only slightly more than one inch (32 millimeters).

Without a doubt, the smaller size of these heads added to the longevity of the total joints with both PTFE and conventional polyethylene. But, small ball size carried with it the two distinct and serious disadvantages of a decreased range of motion and an increased risk of dislocation.

Over time, hip surgeons had not only accepted those limitations, but had become so indoctrinated in Charnley's methods that the topic of using a larger ball never came up. No one had even discussed the possibility of using a normal-size femoral head for almost a generation.

When it occurred to me that we may have eliminated the very need for small femoral heads with our new crosslinked polyethylene, I was stunned by the implications. Dislocation is a leading complication in total hip replacements when smaller head sizes are used. Recurrent dislocations were a leading reason for reoperation. It was easy to imagine that, with the proper-size ball in the socket, far fewer dislocations of the hip would be likely. A larger ball with a more normal, anatomical design might also provide patients with a substantially better range of motion.

We returned to the lab with a simmering sense of excitement. Without anticipating any advance of this type, we were suddenly on the brink of a potentially wonderful outcome beyond what we had envisioned!

One by one, we carefully tested different femoral head sizes in our hip simulator—starting with the tiny 22-millimeter-diameter heads, up to 32 millimeters, and, finally, a normal-size 44-millimeter head. Again, the results were thrilling: *no detectable wear!*

We were elated. All the testing of our crosslinked polyethylene had been superb. Looking back on our progress, I felt each stage had been deeply gratifying.

- **Zero wear.** Loading this material at walking loads during simulated gait 24/7 for six months, the simulation equivalent of 14 to 15 years of walking, had produced zero wear.
- **Molecular reorientation in particle disease.** We had discovered the mechanism by which the tiny submicron particles were formed, substantiating the concept that the submicron particles arose because of reorientation of the molecules.
- **Proof of concept.** We then established proof of concept that crosslinking prevented the reorientation and, thus, reduced wear.
- **Solution to bone destruction.** Our innovative hip simulator demonstrated that our new material was likely to decrease bone destruction substantially, reduce clinical failure, and, most important, eliminate many reoperations, ultimately prolonging the durability of total hip replacements.
- **Resistance to chips.** Our crosslinked polyethylene proved to be the best plastic material devised in 40 years to survive small chips of metal, ceramic, or bone cement in the joint.
- **Reduction of free radicals.** We had also shown that, by melting crosslinked polyethylene, the free radicals left behind after e-beam radiation were gone.
- **Potential reduction of dislocation and reoperation for recurrent dislocation using larger femoral balls.** Crosslinked polyethylene appeared to allow the use of larger femoral balls, which should decrease dislocation of the hip and thereby reduce the need for reoperations for recurrent episodes of dislocation. Remarkably, using even very large femoral ball diameters (44 millimeters) in the simulator had produced zero wear.

With all these achievements behind us and our testing completed, we believed our crosslinked polyethylene qualified, at last, for the ultimate—and most critical—experiment: use in humans.

The possibilities of human application, of course, only led to more questions:

- Among orthopaedic device manufacturers, how many should we choose to make the crosslinked polyethylene? Which one(s) would be best?
- Would it be possible to scale up our benchtop crosslinking technique into an industrial process making millions of pieces? What would it cost?
- What would be the risks to the implant manufacturer if, after being introduced into use in people, the behavior of this new material was different from that in our laboratory studies in terms of wear, deterioration, or, even worse, severe but unanticipated consequences?
- And critically, what position would the FDA take about this material?

We faced the age-old problem of moving from a very promising idea to an actual benefit for humanity. With our combined experience, we had all focused solely on the science of the problem up to this point. Leaving the familiarity and challenges of the laboratory to bring our efforts to fruition in people's lives meant we would have to venture out into strange and unfamiliar new lands.

Our hopes were high. Little did we know what the future would hold.

PART II

Final Hurdles

Victory is reserved for those
who are willing to pay its price.

—SUN TZU

Chapter 11

Terra Incognita: Here Be Dragons!

I am among those who think that science has great beauty.
A scientist in his laboratory is not only a technician; he is also
a child placed before natural phenomena that impress him like a
fairy tale.

— MARIE CURIE, *the only Nobel Prize winner*
in two sciences (Chemistry and Physics)
and the first female Nobel Prize winner

To convert the breakthrough we had created on a small scale in our laboratory into large-scale manufacturing of a product that a company would sell worldwide, we were forced to venture beyond the familiar medical laboratories where each of us had spent the majority of our lives honing our skills, refining our expertise, and building our reputations as clinician–scientists and scientists into a world unknown: terra incognita. There, accompanied by an ever-growing cadre of attorneys and advisors, we would come to fight dragons of a completely different nature than any we had faced before.

With the onslaught of patent applications, nondisclosure agreements (NDAs), FDA applications, challenges from competitors, unexpected lawsuits, and extended manufacturing negotiations, it took far more time to bring the benefits of our new material to patients than it had taken to solve the problem in the first place!

Because I held the erroneous idea that one had to have proof of concept before applying for a patent, we did not apply for patent protection on our crosslinked polyethylene until 1998. Two or three years into that serpentine venture, experience taught us that obtaining a patent is a prolonged, extensive, expensive, multifaceted exercise that must be initiated early. For me, the first shocker was that proof of concept played absolutely no role whatsoever in obtaining a patent. The entire process was so mind-boggling and took so long that, I (somewhat) facetiously posted a new rule on the laboratory wall as a warning to all those who might enter:

IF YOU CONCEIVE AN ORIGINAL IDEA IN THE MORNING, FILE THE
PATENT THAT AFTERNOON.

The premise of patent applications is fundamentally different from that of medical research. From the moment I encountered the inexplicable bone destruction around the hip prosthesis, I was fully engaged in the science of solving its mystery. As I followed the trail, each question we answered raised another one. How could there be bone destruction from macrophages when macrophages can't destroy bone? If bone cement was causing particle disease, why was the disease still thriving in cases without cement? Could polymer science prevent the alignment of polyethylene strands, which was increasing the wear?

In an effort to prove our concept, our research had ranged from designing the first precision hip simulator, to establishing a hypothesis of the wear mechanism, and finally to inventing a crosslinked polyethylene that produced zero wear in the simulator. Until we had solved each one of those mysteries and had in hand a product that was proved to work in the simulator, I had assumed we had nothing to patent. How little I understood the alien world of patent law! There, the goal is to be the first to lay claim to an *idea, not the product*—regardless of whether the idea is life-saving or ridiculous.

The US Patent and Trademark Office is literally buried in applications. It received 618,330 in 2014 alone. With 9500 employees, the Patent Office has a backlog of one million applications. If patent filings stopped today, it would still take the agency two years to catch up. The Patent Office doesn't have time to examine patents for viability. As a result, approved patents range from Benjamin Oppenheimer's emergency fire escape based on a parachute hat, to Toshiba's partially developed seawater desalination system, to Pfizer's recently expired patent for Lipitor, the cholesterol-lowering drug that proved to be the most profitable patent in history.

An entire book could be written about our case alone on the intricacies of patent application and the presentation of claims. This whole essential, prolonged, complicated, and obtuse process was yet one more unanticipated, complex learning experience compelled by our desire to defeat the disease of bone destruction.

Therefore, it was particularly alarming to discover that Harry McKellop and his group in California had been experimenting with crosslinked polyethylene for total hip replacements as well. Although they were using gamma radiation, rather than e-beam radiation, and applying different amounts of radiation, the similarity raised several critical questions: Who originally came up with the concept of crosslinked polyethylene for this medical use?

We were appalled to think that all our labor to this point might be thwarted by having waited so long to file for a patent. Along with our attorneys, we were rightly concerned that the outcome of a decision on that issue could preempt our patent application, not to mention our negotiations with the manufacturing industry. Fortunately, in the long term, both processes for crosslinking polyethylene received patent protection.

Pursuing the patent required an endless series of negotiations with the Patent Office over modification of claims and countless alterations in the application, known as *splits* or *continuations*. It was not just a matter of spending months in a grueling, repetitive, bureaucratic limbo. The real-life experience was that despite filing our patent application in 1998, the patent was not finally granted until *16 years later* in 2014! Fortunately, just the active pursuit of the patent provided us with a substantial amount of protection, even before the patent was awarded, so we were able to approach manufacturers while we waited.

However, before we could reveal any of our ideas to a manufacturer, we had to have protection that the release of our ideas to manufacturers for their consideration would not compromise its secrecy if, in the end, they chose not to sign a licensing agreement. These agreements are called *nondisclosure agreements*, or *NDAs*. When we sought legal counsel that specialized in intellectual property, we immediately hit a snag. To avoid the very important issue of conflict of interest within a legal firm, we could not hire one that had any interaction that could lead to a conflict of interest with either the MGH or MIT. The myriad legal entanglements resulting from the size and complexity of these two huge institutions had created their own cottage industry. Not a single firm dealing with patent law in all of Boston was free of potential conflict of interest. Even more startling, nor were any in New York City, 200 miles away. We were forced to look for counsel in Washington, DC. Our new Washington patent attorneys advised us on both patent protection and NDAs.

But actually, as it came time to approach industry, we uncovered wide differences within our research group about how many manufacturers to involve. One among our inventor group felt strongly that this new material was important enough that it should be made readily available to all patients, and thus to *all* manufacturers. If every patient was to get it, every manufacturer needed to make it. This position had a very compelling moral appeal.

Others pointed out that we should invite as many manufacturers as could be induced to participate. And still others felt a single one would have the largest guarantee of exclusivity to justify the huge investment required to reproduce all our studies, support the processes of getting FDA approval, scale up the manufacturing, and establish worldwide distribution and sales efforts. The FDA approval would be particularly important because FDA submissions of specific implant designs are virtually always done by the manufacturer, and only with clear rights from the FDA to market the product would a manufacturer be willing to move forward. How could we resolve these conflicts about how many manufacturers to involve?

Our resolution benefited from the skill and wisdom of Lita Nelsen, the director of MIT's Technology Licensing Office (Profile 11.1). In the face of our profound ignorance in the realm of patents, licensing, and relationships to industry, Lita's advice was pivotal. Her years of experience in directing the outstanding licensing efforts of guiding the immense inventive output of MIT into successful commercial arrangements were truly invaluable to us.

When we explained our conundrum between making our new material widely available versus giving exclusive rights to a single manufacturer, Lita gave us two pieces of sage advice. Although she confirmed that, based on her experience, no manufacturer would assume the risk of such a massive project without a strong degree of exclusivity, she vigorously advised against aligning with a single manufacturer.

This was because, she explained, after a license had been awarded to a company, we no longer had any say in directing events thereafter. The company would be fully in charge of the

PROFILE 11.1 Lita Nelsen

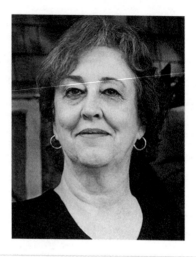

Image courtesy of and reprinted with permission by Lita Nelsen.

Lita Nelsen directs the Technology Licensing Office (TLO) at the Massachusetts Institute of Technology (MIT), which manages more than 300 new inventions annually from three institutions: MIT, the Whitehead Institute, and Lincoln Laboratory. The TLO typically negotiates more than 100 licenses and 20 start-up companies a year.

Lita's *link* to this project was as the director of the TLO, but her *understanding* of the project was quite special. She arrived at MIT on a national scholarship in 1960, and the following summer she had a summer secretarial job at, of all places, MIT, in the chemical engineering department. That fall she took her first course in chemical engineering under Professor Ed Merrill, leading to her bachelor's of science degree thesis under his supervision, followed by becoming a teaching assistant for him while getting her master's degree in chemical engineering.

Lita's first job was, appropriately, with a start-up, Amicon, which developed the field of ultrafiltration. Then followed work at both Arthur D. Little and Millipore Corporation, during which time she achieved an additional master's of science degree in management science.

Lita describes MIT's approach to technology transfer as emphasizing "attracting companies to invest in developing inventions toward commercialization *for the public good*" (emphasis added). While putting a premium on efficient deal making rather than maximizing income, "we seek to maximize the number of inventions licensed to competent companies, with the resulting impact on economic development and public health." This concept has become a model for technology licensing around the world, and Lita has given lectures and seminars on her work in more than 25 countries.

She has also been recognized for this work by receiving the Bayh-Dole Award from the Association of University Technology Managers, and the Lifetime Achievement Award from Global University Ventures. And, amazingly, she is a member of the Excellent Order of the British Empire, MBA (Honorary because she is not a UK citizen).

In addition to advising the National Institutes of Health, the National Academy of Sciences, and the Office of Technology Assessment, she is also the intellectual property advisor to the International AIDS Vaccine Initiative, and a Fellow of the American Institute for Medical and Biological Engineering.

fate of the concept. If they chose not to pursue it at all, we could do nothing about it.

Although it was remotely possible that a manufacturer might deliberately buy a license to squelch a concept, failure to market our product was far more likely to be the result of personnel changes. A new CEO might have less interest in a project. Or, between licensing and production, management might face new economic challenges, develop a different set of priorities, or simply alter the anticipated time schedule. As long as the company made small regular payments (called *minimums*) to the MGH and MIT, the company that owned our license had full rights to stifle the development of this material completely. "Therefore," Lita advised, "always license two companies to provide both an alternative and some competition." If the crosslinked polyethylene proved to be successful, competition between major manufacturers would clearly be valuable to us at every stage. It could accelerate the scale-up process, stimulate the necessary research within the company, and boost enthusiasm for marketing efforts.

Based on this sound advice, we approached not one, but two, major orthopaedic device manufacturers. For reasons of size and geographic diversity, we chose Zimmer, Inc., one of the largest orthopaedic manufacturers in North America, and Sulzer, the largest manufacturer in Europe.

On so many levels, we were embarking on another entirely fresh adventure in forming a relationship with industry. Still, compared with unraveling the mysteries of this previously unknown bone disease that was destroying the hips in more than a million patients around the world, approaching manufacturers appeared fairly simple and straightforward.

Then our FDA consultant provided us with startling news that completely reversed our plans and changed everything.

Like most people, we'd understood that FDA approval was always requested by the manufacturers. However, it was a little known fact that, buried in the 1906 legislation that created the FDA (the Pure Food and Drugs Act) was a pathway for innovators to submit to the FDA themselves! Personally, I was delighted by the news.

When I embarked on this uncertain adventure in 1990, I was 63 years old. I had already had a long and respected career. At the end of that career, I was willing to accept the possibility that I might never succeed in building a no-wear material for total hip joints; but, at the pinnacle of my professional life, the very last thing I wanted was to do something that would harm patients. This was no idle concern, because harming large numbers of patients was exactly what had happened with all three of the prior attempts to improve polyethylene (black poly, heat-pressed poly, and Hylamer) by three of the largest orthopaedic manufacturers in the country.

Our research had been rigorous and our laboratory results spectacularly successful, but FDA approval was known to be an extremely high bar. Our work would be subjected to very stringent criticism by knowledgeable, independent experts whose job was to protect the citizens of the United States. To pass close scrutiny from the serious examination of our crosslinked polyethylene by this expert panel would substantially increase our likelihood of generating safe, long-term outcomes. For me, such a challenge would be invaluable.

Also, one of our basic tenets in approaching any device manufacturer was that the greater the proof of our material and the greater the acceptance that we could generate in the orthopaedic community, the stronger our negotiating power would be. If we approached a manufacturer with nothing but a rough sketch on the back of a napkin, our negotiating position would be limp.

Conversely, if we brought a fully developed physical product, supplemented by excellent research and a strong indication of interest by the FDA, our negotiating position would be strengthened immeasurably.

Seeking FDA approval ourselves allowed us to address both of these vital issues at the same time. We were all enthusiastic about the prospect.

Then the FDA consultant let the other shoe drop.

The innovator pathway, he told us, had virtually never been used. As a result, the FDA had just announced they were closing the pathway—*in just 30 days!* If we wanted FDA evaluation, we would have to complete the complex and intricate FDA application in record time.

Chapter 12

Suddenly, to the FDA

The scientific man does not aim at an immediate result. He
does not expect that his advanced ideas will be readily taken up.
His work is like that of a planter—for the future. His duty is to lay
the foundation of those who are to come and point the way.

—NIKOLA TESLA

We are always very busy in my laboratory at the MGH, but we set new speed records in the 30 days before the inventor pathway to address the FDA was closed. The FDA submission process is demanding and cumbersome. New research and analysis are required. The results must be prepared along very specific lines unique to the FDA. As a result, it's not uncommon for people to take months to fulfill the requirements of the application alone.

To qualify for independent submission before the 30-day window closed, we had to burn a lot of midnight oil. We squeezed every minute we could out of the time allotted. Even FedEx delivery would mean losing a day, so we fell back on an old, but invaluable, trick. On the day of the filing deadline, we flew a team member to Washington to hand deliver our submission in person—just in the nick of time.

Safety and efficacy are the two main concerns of the FDA. Both are tough, but safety is tougher. The key reason is that human experience *always* differs from laboratory testing. Before any human trial starts, it is necessary to speculate about just how different that experience will be from the laboratory tests. No matter how extensive the laboratory testing of a new drug or implant, the human response is always infinitely more complex. It is impossible to replicate fully *outside* the body the conditions that exist *inside* the body.

This creates a certain tension with the release of every new material, device, or drug. The FDA wisely proceeds with caution. Phase 1 of drug testing assesses safety alone by giving a new drug to healthy human volunteers. But the precautions of Phase 1, which are so useful in evaluating new drugs, simply don't apply to devices. Obviously, no one would volunteer to have their normal hip replaced by an artificial hip just to see if the material and/or design were safe.

Consequently, during the evaluation of devices, the FDA relies heavily on prior human experience, even without Phase 1 testing, because patient safety is the main goal. But, if they approve a device, a greater burden falls on the manufacturer, because of the lack of specific prior human testing of this given device. Despite all the successful laboratory tests, severe and devastating failures can and do occur, potentially harming thousands.

Eager to avoid that outcome, the FDA looks for the use of predicate devices. Much like an attorney citing legal precedents, the scientists submitting their applications provide the FDA with examples of somewhat similar materials or designs that have been used previously in patients without adverse effects. Even then, an unavoidable gap exists between the likelihood that the new device will succeed based on the best information available and the unknowns of an actual human trial, if for no other reason than "similar" is not the same as "identical."

We were lucky enough to find three previous human trials with crosslinked polyethylene in total hip surgery. They were all different from ours in important ways.

- **No FDA scrutiny.** Because these human trials occurred in South Africa, Japan, and Great Britain, none had been subjected to FDA scrutiny.
- **No e-beam irradiation.** The polyethylene was crosslinked with gamma radiation in two implants. The third trial used such a strong chemical compound to create the crosslinks that it would have been highly unlikely to get FDA approval.
- **No serious problems for up to 20 years in one case.** Crosslinked polyethylene in these devices was implanted in a relatively small number of patients but, in one instance, for durations up to 20 years without reports of catastrophe or failure. All had shown favorable wear. None had been terminated because of adverse human reactions.
- **Limited knowledge of particle disease.** Crosslinked polyethylene had been chosen for these implants because of its use in industry. The designers had no knowledge of the crucial reorientation of the amorphous strands that led to wear or of particle ingestion by macrophages. Even without understanding these problems, all three implants had shown decreased wear.

Although all three of these devices had been abandoned for other reasons long before we presented our proposal to the FDA, they were meaningful to the FDA nonetheless. None had been abandoned because of material failure. Each one had provided evidence that, even in human trials that spanned as long as two decades in one case, those crosslinked polyethylenes did improve wear. Although we had seen zero wear in the lab in our 14-plus years of simulation, these three trials in humans gave us exactly the kind of evidence we were hoping for!

After the FDA studied our submission, they invited us to a one-hour meeting with their panel of experts. When we arrived, we were quite pleased to see one of their senior officials, who did not often appear during these working sessions, in attendance. It seemed to bode well.

The panel was extremely knowledgeable and asked many penetrating questions. Fortunately, our research had been so extensive that we were readily able to answer nearly all their questions. Things were going so smoothly that the time flew by. It was evident they had considerable interest in our work. Our explanations seemed to satisfy them even more.

As the end of the hour approached, Orhun and I exchanged a tentative smile. Any concerns we had about major resistance by the FDA to our concepts were diminishing. We were just about to launch into our summary and then hear their all-important preliminary response when every alarm bell in every hallway of the building erupted. There was a bomb threat!

Instantly, the enormous building emptied, as people abruptly stopped what they were doing and spilled out onto a grassy field nearby. Teams of firemen rushed into the building to investigate the threat.

This event completely disrupted *the* big moment we'd been anticipating. With much consternation, we found ourselves in the middle of an empty field. We had so many years of hard work invested in the outcome of this presentation that this screeching interruption was disconcerting, to say the least.

And then the senior official strolled over to us on the grass. "I'm quite interested in your idea," he began. "The supporting data are impressive."

"Thank you," I said, shaking his hand.

"It's unofficial, of course, and totally against protocol," he grinned. "But under the circumstances, I suggest we reconvene while we're waiting for the building to be cleared."

We happily agreed. Then, Orhun and I sat down with the members of the FDA panel at a fortuitously located picnic table in the field and continued our discussion.

Although the fire brigade eventually designated the threat a bomb scare, it gave us the unique opportunity to discuss our submission with the panel for an additional hour! During that time, they asked for more data on a variety of conditions we had not yet tested, but they made it clear they would like to consider our ideas and our data. Back in Boston, we quickly generated the additional information they requested and fully alleviated their concerns.

Their interest in our concept was extremely reassuring but had to be considered limited for one specific reason. The FDA only approves *specific devices*, not materials. Therefore, our next step had to be to convince one or more manufacturers to assume the substantial risk and expense of obtaining FDA approval for the specific devices.

Still, the FDA response was remarkably encouraging. FDA approval would be essential in marketing any device in the United States and around the world.

We were, at long last, ready to approach industry.

After the enthusiastic welcome we'd received at the FDA, imagine our surprise to be met with deep skepticism from manufacturers! They still remained extremely negative because of the gross failure of the three previous attempts by three major US manufacturers to reduce the wear of polyethylene.

Among the orthopaedic implant manufacturers, our first two choices were Zimmer, one of the largest US companies, and Sulzer Medical Technology, the largest European company. To our dismay, with a paucity of enthusiasm, Zimmer haltingly carried out protracted negotiations with us. Similarly, Sulzer seemed just as reluctant to entertain the idea of a low-wear polyethylene, particularly because they were the world leaders at that time in the development of metal-on-metal total hips—with the exception of one person. That exception, however, proved crucial.

Urs Wyss, a Swiss engineer who had been a professor of engineering at Queen's University, Kingston, Ontario, had just returned to Sulzer to direct their research program. His knowledge of polymer chemistry—specifically, polyethylene—allowed him to appreciate instantly the remarkable potential of our e-beam crosslinked material (Profile 12.1).

Wyss engaged enthusiastically in his own extensive and independent testing of our material in the labs at Sulzer. Then, from his position of leadership in the company as the head of research, he highly recommended it to Sulzer. His opinion was so well regarded that he completely turned Sulzer around. Instead of indifferent interest, they suddenly evinced a strong desire to bring our product rapidly to market. We signed a licensing agreement.

Despite the testing that had already been done, Sulzer still needed to generate all its own data for every feature of our crosslinked polyethylene. It would not only authenticate our work, but also this was a standard requirement for FDA approval. Simultaneously, Sulzer began extensive efforts to scale up for mass production. We had, of course, warned them about our experience with melting, fires, and explosions in our early studies, and Sulzer's scientists took appropriate precautions while moving swiftly ahead.

Zimmer, on the other hand, continued to procrastinate.

As eager as we were to have two major licensees, and specifically one in the United States and one in Europe, we finally felt compelled to initiate negotiations with a third company, Johnson & Johnson, in part because it was US based. Johnson & Johnson

PROFILE 12.1 Urs Wyss

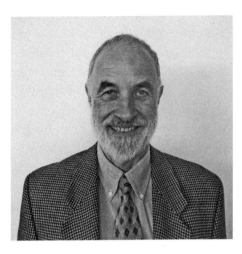

Image courtesy of and reprinted with permission by Professor Urs Wyss.

Urs Wyss was born in 1951 in Bern, Switzerland, and was brought up under simple circumstances. From the beginning, his parents taught him to treat others as he would want to be treated, and they gave him a strong work ethic.

Starting out as a mechanical engineer, Wyss pursued a path to research and development jobs in industry. After considering a medical degree, he decided to build on his engineering background with biomedical skills, ultimately achieving a PhD in biomedicine from the University of Saskatchewan.

During the early 1980s, Wyss joined Sulzer Medical Technology as the first in-house research and development engineer. At the time, Sulzer was the largest manufacturer of artificial joints in Europe.

Wyss coordinated the design of special prostheses for difficult revision operations and for repair after removal of bone tumors. He observed, first hand, the marked difficulty in revision operations caused by substantial bone loss resulting from the wear of polyethylene.

Subsequently, Wyss joined the faculty in mechanical engineering at Queens University in Kingston, Canada, and became the head of that department. There, he pursued numerous research projects in bioengineering and artificial joints with excellent masters and doctoral students at the university. He was introduced to me by Dr. Charles Sorbie, who was the chief of orthopaedic surgery at Queens University.

When Wyss became vice president of research at Sulzer Orthopaedics in Switzerland, he felt lucky to be "at the right place at the right time." They did the very exciting work that led to the commercial introduction of the e-beam crosslinked polyethylene invented in the Harris Laboratory for total hips and in total knees. He considers this to be his best work experience from both the professional and the human points of view.

is a household name in America—not only for pharmaceuticals, but also for medical devices.

We knew their sales of total hip implants were substantially less than those of total knee implants. Nevertheless, they demonstrated distinctly more interest in our material than any other US company. And their very strong total knee program allowed us to entertain the hope that our material might prove to be invaluable in total knee reconstructions as well. Still, this was only a hypothetical possibility, because we had not yet even started any experiments with crosslinked polyethylene for total knee replacements.

With Sulzer rapidly approaching worldwide release of e-beam crosslinked polyethylene, Johnson & Johnson was highly motivated. They agreed to meet with us to sign the license on a Monday.

Three days earlier, on Friday, that plan was thrown into chaos when Zimmer suddenly offered to sign the license instead.

The pressure was on. With particle disease being the number-one cause of total hip replacement failure, every other major orthopaedic manufacturer was now deeply involved in frantic efforts to reduce polyethylene wear. DePuy, another manufacturer, had already licensed the partially crosslinked polyethylene we had learned of when we first pursued a patent.

All in all, it was agonizing weekend of decision making.

Ultimately, based on their stronger total hip program, Zimmer got the nod. And thus, we reached our original ideal: one major US manufacturer and one major European manufacturer. We breathed a great sigh of relief and anticipated smooth sailing from then on.

We should have known better.

Chapter 13

A Regrettable Diversion

*Every new discovery in science brings with it
a host of new problems ....*

—BANESH HOFFMAN

"It knocked my socks off!" my dad used to say. Indeed, it knocked my socks off when we were served notice that *we were being sued!*

A PhD student in chemical engineering, who was working in Ed Merrill's lab at MIT on a totally different and unrelated project was claiming that he had invented e-beam crosslinked polyethylene himself.

We were astonished, but Ed was flabbergasted.

For one thing, virtually everything we did in developing crosslinked polyethylene had been done in the Harris Lab at the MGH. The plaintiff, whom I'll call Kashif, had only been to my lab twice in his life—for 2 hours 15 minutes total—and only as a visitor.

Although we had used MIT equipment to do the radiation of the experimental pieces and for a few quantification measurements, Kashif had had absolutely nothing to do with these or any other steps in our research. He had played no role at all in any aspects of our research at either MGH or MIT.

Why he focused his lawsuit on our project was a complete mystery. My own interactions with him had been minimal, to say the least. On the first occasion, he accompanied Professor

Merrill on a 15-minute sightseeing tour of the lab. Professor Merrill had introduced him to me as a student working on a completely different project. We exchanged brief pleasantries. Nothing more. Several months later, Professor Merrill asked to bring Kashif to one of our weekly project review and planning sessions. It was not an uncommon request. Most graduate students actively take an interest in projects under the supervision of their mentor, even if these other projects are unrelated to their own work. I readily agreed.

That was the scope of my entire interaction with Kashif. Yet somehow he had taken the mind-boggling leap from these two fleeting encounters with our work in the Harris Lab to a claim that he *invented* crosslinked polyethylene! I was furious.

When we got over our astonishment, we quickly assumed we had nothing to worry about. First, he had absolutely no evidence whatsoever to support this preposterous claim. Second, we knew that all employment contracts at both the MGH and MIT transferred ownership of all inventions derived at those institutions directly to those institutions. We *had* actually invented crosslinked polyethylene, but we didn't own it either! Those rights were automatically transferred to MIT and the MGH.

Therefore, this issue looked relatively straightforward to us. On the contrary, this was only a brief prelude of common sense before we descended into a nightmare in which a frivolous lawsuit would disrupt our work for *seven long years* and cost us more than *one million dollars.*

The stakes could not have been higher. If we lost the case, it would be catastrophic for our negotiations with industry. We could lose not only the inventorship, but also MIT and the MGH would lose ownership of the patent.

To defend our case, the MGH administration chose a noted Boston attorney, Fran Lynch (Profile 13.1), who admonished us

PROFILE 13.1 Fran Lynch

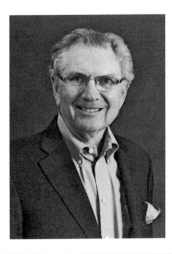

Image courtesy of and reprint permission provided by Marcy Stuart of Marcy Stuart Photography, Auburndale, MA.

After graduating *summa cum laude* from Boston College in 1966 and from Yale Law school in 1969, Fran began his legal practice in an unlikely location: at Rosebud Legal Services in Rosebud, South Dakota. He then returned to Boston, working criminal defense and civil rights cases while also serving as commissioner of the Massachusetts Commission Against Discrimination. After joining Palmer and Dodge in 1978, Fran served as lead counsel in numerous civil cases concerning product liability and trade secrets. During this time, he first represented MIT.

When Fran was hired to respond to the challenge of our inventorship and ownership of our cross-linked polyethylene, he focused his litigation practice on patent cases, including representing MIT, Pharmachemie B.V., and Teva Pharmaceuticals USA. His litigation approach was based on a combination of a nuanced understanding of the legal issues and a detailed familiarity with the specific issues in each case. His extensive understanding of the chemical engineering, biological, and medical aspects of our case enabled him to carry out the vital function of educating Judge Nancy Gertner effectively to the intricacies of the pivotal considerations in this challenge.

In addition to receiving many awards, Fran has been listed in *Who's Who in American Law* since 1983 and in *Who's Who in America* since 1996.

again and again that one can never anticipate the outcome of a court case. Our fate, quite literally, hung in the balance.

We were being forced to invest massive amounts of time and effort to defend our hard work against a graduate student who had contributed nothing. The entire process generated a surprising range of emotions—apprehension, anger, and frustration—as well as an enormous sense of dislocation.

Particularly galling was the profound disruption to our work! After the havoc that bone destruction had been wreaking in the lives of our patients, our crosslinked polyethylene had finally begun to look like a resplendent solution—only to be interrupted by utter legal nonsense.

The very thought that all the years of intense, creative, prolonged efforts that had been invested in this possible solution were being waylaid magnified our anger exponentially. It was especially upsetting to learn the case could not be dismissed out of hand based on the ownership rights of the MGH and MIT because of a technicality, a purported "mistake" made by Kashif in signing the patent transfer paper for MIT. Because he had signed the form at the *top* of the page, not the bottom, he had, technically, not agreed to the conditions. Whether his mistake had been inadvertent or deliberate made no difference to the court. The lack of a correct signature carried legal weight. A second error had been made by the administrator assigned to monitor all signature pages who failed to note and correct this error, but, alas, that made no difference either.

Kashif's claim was based on the issue that he, and he alone, was alerted to the risks of oxidation of highly crosslinked polyethylene and had recommended the methods of eliminating these risks. He claimed that both were unknown to us prior to his suggestion and were essential to the success of the process.

In our minds, this was easily refuted, because Professor Merrill had already published a textbook describing all these aspects of crosslinking years before. Moreover, in my own files was an article on this specific subject that I had read, underlined, and saved, well in advance of Kashif's claim.

In short, not only had he nothing to do with our project, but also he had nothing to do with any research on oxidation whatsoever. No matter what advice he imagined giving us, we had already had intimate knowledge of all these issues long before he arrived. He had made no contribution to our efforts. His claim of inventorship was a sham. Regardless of this fact, it would become excruciatingly clear to us during the next several years that the wheels of justice do, indeed, move slowly.

Before the end, we would learn more about the complexities of the law than we had ever wished to know. We also learned first-hand the remarkable role of good lawyers as extraordinary teachers and students.

For example, in preparing the case, Fran had not only to master the intricacies of human bone destruction by osteoclasts, the role of macrophages, and the details of crosslinking, but also had to condense and articulate these complex subjects brilliantly in lucid ways. All of that sophisticated biochemistry and medical information had to be conveyed succinctly and clearly to a judge or jury. In this regard, as in so many others, Fran Lynch was spectacular.

He and his people "invaded" our laboratory, politely but thoroughly and efficiently. We watched with amazement as they rifled through our files, mastered the pertinent scientific literature, comprehended the nuances of the difficult and sophisticated interrelationships, and identified the exact timing of old and new knowledge. In the end, I had to admit, they actually knew more about the Harris Laboratory than I did!

All of these efforts contributed to the seemingly endless duration of trial preparations. Not only did we carefully discuss the pros and cons of such cases if held in state versus federal courts, but also we pondered whether to pursue a trial with a judge alone or a jury.

Just as all of this was starting to feel like a slow slog through molasses, we discovered that the fact-finding process was even slower.

Depositions, although deliberate and time-consuming, added their own complications. Initially, we faced a well-known, highly successful plaintiff's attorney with a reputation for winning cases for impecunious, downtrodden foreigners being "ripped off" by big institutions in the Boston area, such as MIT and the MGH, which he characterized as heartless, overpowering, and dominating.

Moreover, the entire discovery process had to restart from scratch, not once, but twice, because the plaintiff's attorney changed law firms. To the uninitiated, changing law firms does not appear to be a problem; yet, it easily became an insurmountable issue if the new law firm had potential conflicts of interest with MIT or the MGH, as they did in both instances. As a result, a fresh group of lawyers from a completely different firm took over prosecution of Kashif's claim. Again, not once, but twice.

And if that wasn't enough, the judge who had been initially assigned to the case also had to be changed. When we finally did reach federal court, our case was heard by Judge Nancy Gertner at the John J. Moakley Federal Courthouse at Fan Pier in Boston.

To our complete astonishment, this third team of newcomer attorneys opened the proceedings with an astounding plea—a plea to dismiss the case! Even more surprisingly, that plea was rejected by the judge. After we had struggled with this case for so many years, the issue needed finally to be resolved, she said, once and for all.

After five and one-half long years of discovery, the trial was over in three weeks.

Particularly damning was Kashif's secret recording of a phone call he'd made to Professor Merrill to discuss the lawsuit. When he gleefully submitted the recording to the court as validation of his claims, his error was made plain for all to hear. Ed's comments during the call were patently bland and noncommittal, yet Kashif had twisted his words, to hear what he wanted to hear. We could have hardly offered better evidence ourselves of his distorted, self-serving perspective.

Despite the seriousness of the case and the high stakes riding on its outcome, the trial itself was not without inadvertent humor. Before I took the witness stand, our attorneys introduced me to the court. As is customary, I had been characterized as a paragon of virtue—enormously talented and virtually without blemish. Also, as traditional, it behooved the plaintiff's lawyer to destroy that impression immediately. He did effectively with his very first question.

Presenting me with the typewritten draft of an 18-page paper I had published more than 10 years earlier, he pointed to an editorial note I'd written in the margin on page 10. "Would you please read this note for us?"

I could only stammer. Two things in my life had contributed heavily to the illegible scrawls in the margin that I purported to represent as writing. The first was an occupational hazard: the severe destruction of my penmanship brought on by the furious, unrelenting scribbling of notes during the four years of medical school. The other was my habit of doing the necessary daily editing of manuscripts at the end of the day—usually between 11 PM and midnight—after a very long day of operating, seeing patients, and running experiments in the lab. Although I could not help but feel these were good explanations, I was embarrassed and humiliated that I could not read my own writing.

"Take your time," the attorney said, courteously twisting the knife.

"You have to understand that this was written late at night 10 years ago," I offered. "And besides, I have two excellent secretaries who are paid really well to translate my chicken scratches." It did seem painfully incongruous that this "paragon without blemishes" could not read his own notes.

Question two was worse.

"Let me call your attention to the note in the margin on page 15," the opposing counsel continued. "It appears to be the word 'serendipity.' Is that correct?"

Relieved to be able to read it, I felt the blush leave my skin. "Yes, that's correct."

"Can you also acknowledge that the word is misspelled?"

Again, the feeling of sharp humiliation. Just as my face was returning to crimson, Judge Gertner intervened. "Counsel," she asked, "you have established that this witness can neither read nor spell. Where are you going with this line of questioning?" He immediately abandoned that line of questioning. If I could have, I would have kissed Judge Gertner on the spot.

Unfortunately, when the trial ended, an unrelated circumstance radically postponed the verdict and created a harrowing period of uncertainty for us. As it happened, Judge Gertner was, simultaneously, in the process of creating a major, national legal position on the issue of mandatory sentencing. That important work delayed her ruling on our case for a very disconcerting 18 months.

The wait proved to be well worth it.

In her 60-page verdict, Judge Gertner sharply criticized Kashif both for filing the lawsuit and for the manner in which he presented his case. This reinforced our suspicions about whether his misplaced signature on the transfer of ownership at MIT had, in fact, been deliberate.

Although we remained deeply dismayed at this enormously painful digression caused by this diversion, we were delighted to be able to move forward once again.

Chapter 14

Unforeseen Complications

When everything seems to be going against you, remember
an airplane takes off against the wind, not with the wind.

— HENRY FORD

Our excitement at reaching this pinnacle was palpable. Looking back, we could see what an amazing constellation of events had taken place. We had blended our work with that of many others to identify a mysterious new disease and determine its causes, developed the first authentic hip simulator, potentially resolved the entire problem of bone destruction with the new crosslinked polyethylene, tested it for wear with extraordinarily successful results, received an enthusiastic response of the FDA—and now came the pivot to industry. The scale-up in the manufacturing world would lay the groundwork for the ultimate test, the only *real* test: human trials.

However, many things can go wrong when a relatively small laboratory process is magnified to a scale sufficient for worldwide distribution. In theory, the same general principles should hold true for a large-scale production as for the pilot processes regardless of scale, but in practice it doesn't always work out that way.

The scale-up by the European company Sulzer worked remarkably well, despite the fact that they modified our protocol to suit their own procedures for generating e-beam radiation.

Strangely enough, the American company, Zimmer, followed our protocol to the letter, yet somehow their socket pieces were at times completely unacceptable, substandard material. Particularly confusing was the fact that certain batches of the Zimmer products came out perfectly whereas others failed completely. How was this possible? Although efforts to resolve this problem were collegial at first, later on, as the resolution remained obscure, tense conversations among the scientists at the MGH, MIT, and Zimmer only made matters worse. Skeptics and naysayers appeared from every direction.

As frustration mounted, Orhun felt he had to see the problem firsthand, at the site of the e-beam irradiation process that Zimmer had selected. He flew across the country to Seattle to watch the scale-up process himself to see whether he noticed anything that no one else had.

Unwittingly, he was following the sage advice of my physician father to "go see the patient." When the reports don't add up, the results are inconsistent, and the reasons seem confusing, go look at the process yourself. As it turned out, that adage applied just as soundly to manufacturing as it did to medicine.

When he was there in person, it took Orhun just minutes to figure out what the problem was. As soon as he walked into the warehouse where the irradiation was taking place, he noticed the technicians were wearing jackets. When he started to take off his own coat, one of them said, "I wouldn't do that, if I were you. It's expected to get down to 45 degrees today!"

"There's no heat in here?" Orhun asked, incredulous.

"Nah, we're used to it," the technician shrugged.

In the lab at MIT, the polyethylene always rested at room temperature at about 70 degrees Fahrenheit before being irradiated with the e-beams. Zimmer was irradiating the plastic in a large, unheated warehouse where the ambient temperature in the winter dropped to 45 degrees Fahrenheit.

The magnitude of the effect of adiabatic heating is very sensitive to changes in the starting temperature of the polyethylene. The different temperature in the warehouse between summer and winter explained why some of Zimmer's production lines were fine and why others failed. The ambient starting temperature made all the difference. After that defect in the manufacturing process was resolved, the crosslinked polyethylene socket pieces came out perfectly acceptable, regardless of the time of year of their manufacture.

Although *that* disturbing impediment to our progress was resolved effectively after considerable consternation and some acrimony, it was quickly overshadowed by an even more obtuse and unsettling problem. Moreover, at first, this new issue did not even appear to have anything to do with us or with our crosslinked polyethylene.

Sulzer suddenly found itself in huge distress.

In an effort to reduce costs, the new president had attempted to shorten the manufacturing process used in making the metal shells to contain the polyethylene. Two outside testing laboratories had validated the new process, but very rapidly the total hip operations done using these new metal shells started failing, and in large numbers

Why? Because the metal shells did not bond to the skeleton. Bone did not grow in. The many failures were severely painful. Regrettably, patients required a reoperation with the insertion of an alternate metal shell. Sulzer was forced to issue a recall for *17,000* of these implants, which put the company in jeopardy. The first few successful court cases against these unacceptable metal shells alone resulted in judgments against Sulzer for many millions of dollars each. Sulzer would not survive many more such judgments.

Desperate, Sulzer took a totally unprecedented step. They hired Richard Scruggs, the *plaintiffs'* attorney made world famous in his successful, high-profile lawsuits against both the asbestos industry and the tobacco industry (Profile 14.1). Because much of Scruggs' past legal work involved class-action suits *against* manufacturers, this was a stunning move on Sulzer's part. It was an equally strange move for Scruggs, such a committed plaintiffs' attorney working against big companies, to take this case in defense of Sulzer. Everyone involved was highly curious about what would happen next.

In a remarkable turn of events, Scruggs, now Sulzer's *defense* attorney, initiated a class-action suit *against* Sulzer! He argued that, if every victim of the implants (which Sulzer already acknowledged were faulty) filed a lawsuit, it would bankrupt the company and no one except the very first few plaintiffs would receive compensation.

In contrast, a class-action settlement would allow the court to distribute awards equitably to *all* those who had been harmed. But for this solution to succeed, Sulzer had to stay in business.

The court reviewed the company's books in detail and assessed a level of compensation that would also permit the company to survive, rather than granting huge, unsustainable settlements to the first few plaintiffs with successful suits. This was a brilliant idea; it kept Sulzer alive but, obviously, severely compromised. Unfortunately, Sulzer was eventually forced into bankruptcy nonetheless, returning under a new name: Centerpulse. It was a smaller, weaker company.

In the final twist to this strange episode, it was then that Zimmer purchased Centerpulse (the former Sulzer)! Of course,

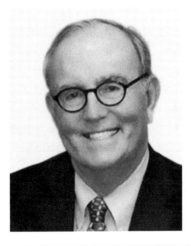

Image courtesy of and reprinted with permission by Richard F. Scruggs.

Scruggs is a former lawyer and Navy fighter pilot. He is best known as the architect of the litigation that resulted in the multibillion dollar Tobacco Settlement, and for later going to federal prison in a judicial bribery scandal. In prison, Dickie taught general educational development (GED) to other inmates. That experience led him, upon his release, to establish Second Chance Mississippi, which is a nonprofit collaborative effort with Mississippi's Community Colleges to raise awareness and funds for GED and adult education.

Dickie is a native Mississippian and an Ole Miss graduate. He and his wife, Diane, have been married 44 years, and moved to Oxford, Mississippi, from the East Coast of the United States in 2003. The Scruggs' have two grown children and four grandchildren, and they are members of the First Presbyterian Church.

this put an end to our careful strategy to license two major manufacturers: one in America and one in Europe.

Following the clearly marked trail that we had blazed at the FDA, both Zimmer and Sulzer–Centerpulse moved vigorously to prepare its own presentation. They sought approval for the specific components they had designed and manufactured using our crosslinked polyethylene. The FDA panel was every bit as enthusiastic about these devices as it had been about the materials we had discussed with them previously during the bomb scare. Their approval activated the next hurdle: use in real people.

As ever, this raised yet the next challenging question: How would we know if our crosslinked polyethylene actually worked in people? How would we determine the success or failure of our material in human beings without waiting 10 to 15 years to find out whether we had eliminated the bone destruction? Stated another way: How could we measure the wear of crosslinked polyethylene *in patients?*

We could no longer measure wear directly as we had done using the hip simulator. Nor could we retrieve specimens for direct measurements during human use unless the total hip failed. So how would we know if the crosslinked polyethylene was working in humans?

Fortunately, two methods of measuring wear of polyethylene in living patients had already been developed. Although very different, they were quite complementary.

The most accurate one goes by another jaw-breaking name— *radiostereometric analysis,* best referred to as *RSA.* Although it seems impossible, RSA can actually measure the wear of polyethylene in the hip joint in patients with an accuracy of about one third the thickness of a human hair—a tiny amount of about 30 microns.

To achieve such miniscule accuracy, multiple tiny metal beads are buried in the pelvic bone and the femur of the patient during the surgery. Although these beads do not damage the bones, they serve as markers for reference in the specialized x-rays that permit not only two-dimensional but also three-dimensional analysis.

Because of the complexity of these RSA techniques, very few laboratories in the world perform RSA studies. In addition, because they were not permitted in the United States by the FDA in 1995, there were no labs in the United States conducting RSA studies. What were we to do?

The second option, known as the *Martell method*, analyzed ordinary x-rays with special techniques. Although it was less accurate than RSA, it had the huge advantage that it was being used on large numbers of patients at multiple orthopaedic centers around the world.

We chose to apply both methods to quantify the wear of our crosslinked polyethylene in patients.

We turned to the world's leading program for RSA studies at Sahlgrenska University in Goteborg, Sweden, under the direction of Peter Herberts and Henrik Malchau (Profile 14.2). We negotiated two RSA studies there: one for the Zimmer version for our crosslinked polyethylene called *Longevity*, and one for the Sulzer version called *Durasul.*

As we knew they would, and to our considerable delight, the Sahlgrenska group brought rigorous standards and an exacting scientific ethos to the studies, as well as the best RSA technique in the world. We needed all these attributes to assess our material most critically.

If somehow our concepts or experiments were wrong or even just incomplete, vast numbers of patients would be at risk. So, we sought a *completely* unbiased outside evaluation and placed a high

PROFILE 14.2 Henrik Malchau

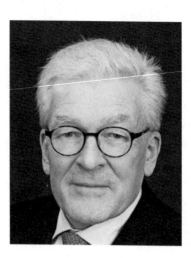

Image courtesy of and reprinted with permission by Professor Henrik Malchau.

Henrik Malchau was born in Saeby, a small town in northern Jutland in Denmark, as the middle of three children. He enrolled in medical school at the University of Aarhus in 1969. During medical school he developed a strong commitment to health care in the Third World. Consequently, he took a one-year sabbatical and worked on a project on prophylactic health care for bushmen in central Kalahari, Botswana. That compelling experience opened his eyes to health care outside of Denmark. After graduating from medical school, he took the specialized graduate examination, which, years later, would allow him to practice medicine in the United States and thus to apply for a position at the Massachusetts General Hospital (MGH) and Harvard Medical School (HMS).

During medical school, Malchau spent summer vacations as an intern in a small hospital in Lysekil, along the Swedish west coast. There he met his wife of 38 years and decided to move to Sweden for his clinical education. His internship and residency were shared between Uddevalla and Sahlgrenska hospitals, and in 1983 he became an attending orthopaedic surgeon at Sahlgrenska University Hospital in Goteborg, Sweden.

With Peter Herberts as mentor, Malchau became involved in the Swedish Hip Arthroplasty Register, where for many years he had a leadership role. This registry collected nationwide information on all total hip arthroplasties (THA) and their subsequent complications in Sweden. He has also acted as an advisor for setting up registries in Australia, Canada, New Zealand, England, and the United States.

Parallel to this, Malchau was also engaged in radiostereometric analysis (RSA) of implant stability and polyethylene wear in THA. These research efforts were summarized in his PhD thesis in 1995, titled "On the Importance of Stepwise Introduction of New Hip Implant Technology."

At the American Academy of Orthopaedic Surgeons meeting in 1996, I made contact with Malchau after a presentation, and that led to a sabbatical year (2000–2001) at the Harris Orthopaedic Laboratory at the MGH. That subsequently led to an invitation to become an attending surgeon at the MGH and ultimately to the role of codirector of the Harris Lab, a joint position with Orhun Muratoglu. During many years in these positions, Malchau has continued his efforts to improve the evidence base for new total joint implants by use of RSA and registries. He was recognized for his efforts by an appointment as full professor at HMS, and subsequently was also granted the Alan Gerry Chair in Orthopaedic Surgery at HMS.

Malchau has published 200 peer-reviewed papers, has been presidential guest lecturer at the US Hip Society twice, and received three Hip Society awards. He is a cofounder of the International Society for Arthroplasty Registries, has been president of the International Hip Society, and is an honorary fellow of the British Hip Society. He has received multiple other national and international awards.

value on their role as independent, objective scientists with no relationship to the development of the material.

As the current century began to unfold, we were just beginning to see firsthand the tragic results of the widespread use of metal-on-metal total hips, despite their strong promise (see Chapter 15), but we were desperate to learn that our crosslinked polyethylene made matters better, not worse. If anything was wrong, we needed to be the first to know it and we needed to know it absolutely as early as possible, specifically at the very first suggestion.

The research team at Sahlgrenska had earned an unquestioned reputation for total integrity and independence in critical research in its use of RSA. Using this technique, they had previously shown definitively that a proposed new bone cement was severely deficient. This, along with several other similar studies, had prevented several worldwide disasters. Moreover, in doing RSA investigations, only small numbers of patients were placed at risk. Their objectivity and excellence had already headed off much larger disasters. In the event that any vulnerability existed in our material, we hoped the Sahlgrenska studies would do the same for us.

During the negotiations to do these studies, Sahlgrenska wanted even more rigorous testing than even we did. For example, they insisted the studies be funded for 10 years, a virtually unheard-of duration in clinical orthopaedic studies. Studies of this length were essential, however, because the bone destruction we were trying to eliminate had taken that long to develop in the past. In December 1998, our first RSA patient entered the study.

Now that we had established two ways to measure wear of our material in living patients, we faced the final two, and ultimately dominating, questions: Would the crosslinked polyethylene eliminate the bone destruction? And was it free of adverse reactions and/or failure mechanisms? Both these questions would take many years to assess. But, these two essential issues came intimately accompanied by a key *surrogate*—specifically, the measurement of *wear* as an indicator of whether it was likely or predictable that both ultimate aims would be reached.

Our hopes were pinned on the RSA and Martell studies both to measure wear as a predictor of bone destruction and to alert us of any early failures, should they occur. We were on the brink of finding out whether we had actually found a way to eliminate bone destruction. The die was cast and we had to await the outcome. Nine years had passed since we embarked on this adventure, and many more would pass before we would know the answer.

Chapter 15

Panic

If the results confirm the hypothesis, you've made a discovery.
If the result is contrary to the hypotheses, you've made a discovery.

—ENRICO FERMI

While all of these developments for the crosslinked polyethylene were being put in motion and we had begun to implant crosslinked polyethylene in patients at the turn of this century, it happened again: the totally unexpected. Perhaps we should've gotten used to it by then, but can any of us ever really learn to expect the unexpected?

At the start of the new century, isolated reports appeared of a new, very disturbing finding. Extensive, adverse tissue reactions were occurring in patients with metal-on-metal hip replacements: *pseudo-tumors*. Masses of soft tissue were forming around the metal-on-metal prostheses, sometimes accompanied by very aggressive bone destruction. In the famous words of Yogi Berra, "It was *déjà vu* all over again."

In the decades since my initial case with Peter Dunn in 1974, orthopaedic surgeons had been forced to become accustomed to severe cases of bone destruction from the old polyethylene. But, as these pseudo-tumors (i.e., extremely severe reactions to metal-on-metal total hip replacements) continued to appear in alarming numbers after 2000, even experienced surgeons were aghast at the overwhelming, massive destruction in these metal-on-metal cases. It was not only because of the extent of the damage, but also because of a frightening new kind of damage. This form of bad reaction to the metal-on-metal total hip replacements not only "ate" bone, it "ate" muscles and even "ate" nerves. In severe cases, the bones and muscles that enabled the hip joint to move were badly destroyed. Also, the *sciatic nerve*, which is essential to the function of the leg, could be destroyed!

We wondered what on Earth could be causing this horrifying condition, and why had this previously unseen severe reaction emerged for the first time in the 40-year use of metal-on-metal hip replacements?

Skeptics of metal-on-metal total hip replacements had pointed out for decades that an absolutely overwhelming number of very tiny (nano-size) particles were released by metal-on-metal joints. It was true that these particles were even smaller and vastly greater in number than the multitudinous particles that resulted from conventional polyethylene.

Despite that fact, pseudo-tumors had never been a problem— until 2000—they were suddenly widespread and, worse, on the rise. Not only were pseudo-tumors cropping up with metal-on-metal conventional hip replacements, they were also appearing in another form of metal-on-metal total hips, called *surface replacements*, where the natural ball of the patient's hip joint was preserved and covered with a thin metal shell.

Pseudo-tumors were soon revealed to be caused by a severe, adverse tissue reaction to, as was no surprise, "particulate debris." It was particle disease all over again, but now in a new and extreme form: metal particles.

The mystifying question was, why had this phenomenon not been observed during the previous 40 years of metal-on-metal total hip replacements? The answer to that question remains a mystery even today. It may be explained in part by the fact that, during the 1960s and 1970s, most metal-on-metal hip replacements had not survived long enough to produce pseudo-tumors, although many others had survived for decades without incident.

By this time, following the turn of this century, the problem had reached crisis proportions. Major newspapers such as *The New York Times* and the *Boston Globe*, ran series of prominent articles on this worldwide medical disaster. In the United States alone, an estimated 650,000 patients had received metal-on-metal total hip replacements. With certain designs, 40% of the implants produced pseudo-tumors in less than 10 years and required reoperation. In another series, destruction occurred in 30% after just six years and climbed to 50% by 10 years.

These high failure rates were compounded by the extraordinary difficulty of repairing the aggressive muscle, nerve, and bone damage. In the most severe cases, repair was virtually impossible. When there was major muscle destruction, dislocation of the hip was very common and even more difficult to repair. In a few extreme examples, ions from the metal particles filled the bloodstream in such high concentrations that patients developed mental and visual abnormalities from *metal ion poisoning*.

Needless to say, use of metal-on-metal prostheses dropped to virtually zero around the world. Every company, except one, withdrew them from the market. Following the strategy developed for Sulzer by Richard Scruggs, class-action suits against the makers of metal-on-metal implants proliferated. The staggering liability cost for several manufacturers was in excess of $1.5 billion, pending further liabilities. Very quickly, the field of "alternate bearings" for total hip replacements narrowed from three candidates to two: metal-against-crosslinked polyethylene or ceramic on ceramic.

But for all of us in my laboratory working on crosslinked polyethylene, our empathy for those patients who now had pseudo-tumors from their metal-on-metal prostheses was heavily compounded by our own apprehensions that some similar unexpected, severe, late-onset adverse reaction to the crosslinked polyethylene might occur. Just before the early and completely unexpected identification of the pseudo-tumors around metal-on-metal total hips, our highly crosslinked polyethylene acetabular component was implanted into our first patient. What might be its fate in actual use in people?

If any problem arose in a patient who had our crosslinked polyethylene that required a reoperation, we would finally have our first chance to retrieve a specimen after human use and investigate the problem. Of course, it was our most profound hope that nothing would go wrong. If it did, we could only hope it would be a long wait.

As we implanted more total hips with our new material, we anticipated being able to analyze the resultant wear on some implants sooner than others. There are inevitable complications following total hip surgery, such as infections or dislocations that might allow us to take a look at the implant even without a material failure. A chance to evaluate one of our hips more closely might have also occurred after an automobile accident or unexpected death from other causes. Regardless of our best efforts to keep our patients healthy and well, opportunities to examine our highly crosslinked polyethylene after human use would surely occur.

When the first specimen did arrive in my laboratory, obtained after a patient had died of causes unrelated to the hip, we were obviously very eager to evaluate its condition. Would there be any changes to the joint surface? What kind of wear would our crosslinked polyethylene produce in the human body, after dazzling us with zero wear in laboratory conditions?

We all rushed to the lab, hoping to find our handiwork perfectly intact. It might be a moment of triumph—the long-awaited validation that had motivated our efforts for decades. Instead, we had a very bad day.

The final stages of manufacturing of the socket pieces produce a beautiful component. The sophisticated machining process creates fresh joint surfaces on each implant with parallel circumferential rows of shallow hills and valleys called *machine marks* (Figure 15.1).

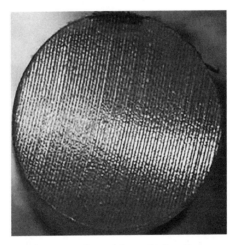

FIGURE 15.1 *Machine Marks on Acetabular Component Before Insertion*

Photograph of a portion of the surface of a highly crosslinked acetabular component before being introduced into a patient. Note the highly regular, parallel ridges and grooves. These are the result of the final machining process and are called *machine marks*.

Instead of seeing what we expected, the formerly pristine surface of the retrieved implant was extremely disfigured, scratched, and gouged. Grooves cut across the machine marks at strange angles, sometimes obliterating the machine marks completely with severe scuffing (Figure 15.2).

This appearance, also, stood in marked contrast to the retrieved specimens of surfaces of conventional polyethylene, where the machine marks on the surface were never visible. Those surfaces were always completely smooth and glistening as a result of the excessive wear.

Looking at the marred surface of our crosslinked polyethylene after human use stoked our worst fears. What had gone wrong? Was this a forerunner of something like what was appearing in the

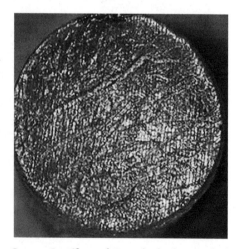

FIGURE 15.2 *Severe Scuffing of Crosslinked Acetabular Component*

Photograph of a crosslinked acetabular component removed after several years' use in a patient. Note the irregular scuffing, scratching, and streaking across the surface, probably indicating extensive damage and wear.

pseudo-tumors of the metal-on-metal hips? Was this evidence of some unseen Achilles heel in our entire process? What were the implications for the durability of the material, for the lifetime of the total hip itself, and for the destructive effects of the wear particles?

The retrieved hip implant specimen was so grooved and gouged it looked as if significant chunks of polyethylene had been ripped out and released into the body. In years to come, as we well knew, this could result in the same devastating particle disease we were desperate to avoid.

With this first specimen, my hopes were dashed completely. It was heartbreaking. After many years of effort, had we actually created a material that produced *more wear?*

Orhun Muratoglu was crestfallen too, but because polymers were his area of expertise, he was immediately engaged in the specific issue of how this could happen. He knew of a number of interactions that might cause this kind of response, but why was it happening so totally unexpectedly here? How could we be misled so completely by our extensive hip simulator studies? Orhun left the room to ponder quietly the range of possible explanations for this bizarre effect.

When he returned, his answer was exhilarating!

Looking at the specimen more closely, Orhun was not convinced that *any* of the polyethylene had been lost. To test his theory, he subjected the polyethylene specimen to heat, enough heat to *melt* it.

Because, as I mentioned before, polyethylene has the remarkable property of shape memory, it remembers its original shape and returns to exactly that shape when it is cooled after it has been melted. Orhun put this principle of shape memory to the test. When he melted and then cooled the "damaged" specimens, *all the original machine marks were fully restored* (Figure 15.3B)!

There were no gaps or missing pieces. No material had been worn away. This could only mean that the grooves and gouges were superficial scuffing.

When Orhun measured the volume of the polyethylene that remained, it was exactly the same as it had been when the hip replacement was new. Nothing had been lost. All the highly crosslinked polyethylene was still there; it was just scuffed up. It was a surface distortion caused by rough patches that commonly develop on the surface of the metal femoral heads or by third bodies that work their way into the joint. So, too, all the

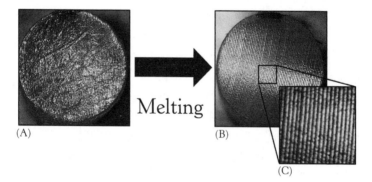

(A)   Melting   (B)

(C)

FIGURE 15.3 *Upon Closer Examination Before and After Melting to Elicit Shape Memory*

Photographs showing the effect of shape memory on the scuffing of the surface of the crosslinked polyethylene. (A) This photo is the same as Figure 15.1, showing the widespread scuffing of the surface during use in a patient. (B) This photo is the identical piece of crosslinked polyethylene after the specimen had been melted and cooled. Melting and cooling restored the polyethylene to its original shape through its shape memory feature. Now it looks exactly like the surface before being inserted in the body. This shows no material was lost and no wear occurred. Scuffing had occurred, distorting the surface, but not wearing it. (C) This photo is a close-up of the surface showing the machine marks after being restored.

subsequent retrieved specimens that we obtained showed this frightening, but actually reinforcing, appearance. During its time in the human body, the surface of the polyethylene had simply been shoved around into a scuffed configuration. *No material had been lost* (Figure 15.3).

The crosslinked polyethylene was intact. We could relax. At least for the time being.

Chapter 16

Ubiquitous Success

Fortune sides with those who dare.

—VIRGIL

To evaluate the impact of our crosslinked polyethylene on reducing wear and decreasing bone destruction, fast-forward 18 years from the time of the first implantation of this material to the present. First, did our crosslinked polyethylene, indeed, reduce wear? The short answer is an emphatic *yes!* The reduction in wear was dramatic, even startling, and ubiquitous.

But, before displaying the evidence that establishes the remarkable success of crosslinked polyethylene in virtually eliminating the disease of bone destruction adjacent to components of total hip replacements, it is important to present an overall perspective of this achievement. Many, many things contributed either in conjunction or in parallel with the development of crosslinked polyethylene. For example, for those surgeons using bone cement, improved techniques of its use have helped substantially. For those using cementless techniques, progressive advances in their design and manufacture have aided considerably. The advances in ceramic-on-ceramic joints, similarly, have been extremely effective in reducing bone destruction. And an alternate form of crosslinked polyethylene, different from ours, is also fully successful.

Still, even within *that* perspective, consider the remarkable worldwide effect of the revolutionary results of crosslinked polyethylene in total hip replacements. A dramatic change in any field is rare, hence the term *breakthrough*. For the first four decades of total hip surgery—in essence, the entire lifetime of total hip surgery before crosslinked polyethylene—the primary material used to replace cartilage was conventional polyethylene, but it had a fatal flaw: wear. Wear led to bone destruction and, thus, for many patients, the total hip replacement, which had initially provided spectacular pain relief and restored remarkable mobility to their lives, became a living nightmare.

For the first time, crosslinking the polyethylene had virtually eliminated polyethylene wear. Astonishingly and effectively, the problem of polyethylene wear had been overcome.

Extensive studies of total hip operations done for patients with many different diagnoses by vastly different surgeons in many different countries with widely different surgical techniques all documented marked reduction in wear again and again and again.

This widespread confirmation of low wear was somewhat like hearing drums in the jungle. When you hear the drums from just one direction, you pay attention, but you are not quite sure what it means. When you hear the drums thrumming from several directions—the east, the west, the north, and then the south—the message carries much more credence. The jungle drums telling of remarkably low wear rates of highly crosslinked polyethylene and of the absence of the destructive bone disease adjacent to the prostheses were beating all over the world.

Data from Sweden and Australia supported the findings from Great Britain and New Zealand, and numerous other countries around the world. All showed excellent results and very low wear and no, or only very rare, bone destruction. Confirmation of the dramatic reduction in wear by crosslinking polyethylene was universal.

Tables 16.1 and 16.2 demonstrate the uniformity of the data using seven different measuring techniques. In the 10-year human studies with high-resolution RSA, the crosslinked polyethylene showed no measurable wear! Compare this with conventional polyethylene, which wore, on average, at a rate of 100 microns or more per year (more than 1000 microns over 10 years). These were stunning results!

The study designs, some of which included randomized controlled experiments, as well as the very high accuracy and resolution of RSA, represented the pinnacle of rigorous science. Because the RSA studies were conducted by the renowned Swedish scientists at Sahlgrenska University, who were the world's leading practitioners of RSA studies, their results were beyond dispute in the medical community.

Nonetheless, there were limits to the RSA studies and, with millions of new patients getting these implants, the stakes were high. Because we wanted to exercise an abundance of caution, we took our testing even further.

The primary limitations of the RSA studies were the small number of patients studied and the fact that they were all Swedes. Less than 30 hips with crosslinked polyethylene and 30 hips with conventional polyethylene had been evaluated over 10 years. Because patients' activities differ by age, country, and culture, as well as the impact of differing indications for surgery by cultural differences and the variations in diseases found in separate countries, a wide mix of subjects is of great value in assessing any new technique or implant. Ideally, we needed data from many more patients of different ages with different diagnoses from all over the world.

TABLE 16.1 Ten-year Results or Longer in Total Hip Replacement in Patients 50 Years or Younger: Wear and Bone Destruction Using Highly Crosslinked Polyethylene

Author	Number of hips	Type of ball	Median age (years)	Wear in microns/ year	Bone destruction
Kim et al. (A)	67	Ceramic	28	31	0
Babovic and Trousdale	54	Metal	39	20	0
Kim et al. (B)	100	Ceramic	44	31	0
Garvin et al.	96	Metal or ceramic	42	22	0

Notes: (A) Kim Y, Park J, Patel C, Kim D. Polyethylene wear and osteolysis after cementless total hip arthroplasty with alumina-on-highly cross-linked polyethylene bearings in patients younger than thirty years of age. *J Bone Joint Surg Am.* 2013; 95: 1088–1093.

Babovic N, Trousdale RT. Total hip arthroplasty using highly cross-linked polyethylene in patients younger than 50 years with minimum 10-year follow-up. *J Arthroplasty.* 2013; 28: 815–817.

(B) Kim Y, Park J, Kulkarni SS, Kim Y. A randomised prospective evaluation of ceramic-on-ceramic and ceramic-on highly cross-linked polyethylene bearings in the same patients with primary cementless total hip arthroplasty. *Int Orthop.* 2013; 37: 2131–2137.

Garvin KL, White TC, Dusad A, Hartman CW, Martell J. Low wear rates seen in THAs with highly crosslinked polyethylene at 9 to 14 years in patients younger than age 50 years. *Clin Orthop Rel Res.* 2015; 473: 3829–3835.

Such a widespread selection was not possible with the RSA technique, so we used the Martell technique in addition. At six hospitals in North America, we studied 768 patients of various ages and ethnicities for 10 years or more. In the end, many patients had no wear at all, and the average wear was found to be just 20 microns per year (about one fifth the thickness of a human hair).

TABLE 16.2 Ten-year Results or Longer in Patients with Average Age Older than 50 Years: Wear and Bone Destruction Using Highly Crosslinked Polyethylene

Author	Number of hips	Type of ball	Median age (years)	Wear in microns/year	Bone destruction
Johanson et al.	25	Metal	55	5	5*
Bedard et al.	150	Metal	56	50	0
Bragdon et al. (A)	174	Metal	60	18	0
Garcia-Rey et al.	45	Metal	67	20	0
Glyn-Jones et al.	39	Metal	68	33	0
Engh et al.	72	Metal	63	40	0
Snir et al.	43	Metal	60	50	2
Bragdon et al. (B)	768	Metal or ceramic	57.1	9	0

Notes: *Calcar bone loss.

Johanson P, Digas G, Herberts P. Highly crosslinked polyethylene does not reduce aseptic loosening in cemented THA: 10-Year findings of a randomized study. *Clin Orthop Rel Res.* 2012; 470(11): 3083–3093.

Bedard NA, Callaghan JJ, Stefl MD, Willman TJ, Liu SS, Goetz DD. Fixation and wear with a contemporary acetabular component and cross-linked polyethylene at minimum 10-year follow-up. *J Arthroplasty.* 2014; 29: 1961–1969.

(A) Bragdon C, Doerner M, Rubash H, et al. Clinical multi-centric studies of the wear performance of highly crosslinked remelted polyethylene in THR. *Clin Orthop Rel Res.* 2013; 471(2): 393–402.

Garcia-Rey E, Garcia-Cimbrelo E, Cruz-Pardos A. New polyethylenes in total hip replacement: A 10-to 12-year follow up study. *Bone Joint J.* 2013; 95: 326–332.

Glyn-Jones S, Geraint ERT, Garfield-Roberts P, et al. Highly crosslinked polyethylene in total hip arthroplasty decreases long-term wear: A double-blind randomized trial. *Clin Orthop Rel Res.* 2015; 473: 432–438.

Engh CA Jr, Hopper RH, Huynh C, Ho H, Sritulanondha S, Engh CA Sr. A prospective, randomized study of cross-linked and non-cross-linked polyethylene for total hip arthroplasty at 10-year follow-up. *J Arthroplasty.* 2012; 27(8): 2–8.

Snir N, Kaye ID, et al. 10-Year follow-up wear analysis of first-generation highly crosslinked polyethylene in primary total hip arthroplasty. *J Arthroplasty.* 2014; 29: 630–633.

(B) Bragdon CR, Barr CJ, Nielsen CS, et al. Minimum 10-year multi-center study of THR with highly cross-linked polyethylene and large diameter femoral heads. Presented at the Hip Society, Dallas TX, November 5–8, 2015.

This rate was well below the threshold of wear that might result in bone destruction. It was dramatically lower than the wear of conventional polyethylene. All these studies showed that wear was eliminated in many patients, and sharply reduced in the rest.

With the massive reduction of polyethylene wear, we had crossed the first threshold in our quest to conquer the bone destruction! Although we were delighted with the reduction in wear, in reality wear was not the true endpoint of our quest. Reduction in the bone destruction was. Decreasing wear might be the key way to prevent bone destruction, but it was, in fact, a surrogate for our real end point: the sharp decrease or elimination of the bone destruction.

What about the heart of the matter: bone destruction near the prosthesis. When we had begun this journey, total hip replacement—one of history's most successful major operations—was dangerously threatened.

The tremendous ability of this operation to free people from pain and restore them to a life of full activity and to overcome crippling disability by lifting people out of their wheelchairs was severely challenged by the particle disease that aggressively destroyed the adjacent bones. Particle disease had actually completely halted the worldwide use of metal-on-metal implants because of the pseudo-tumors that developed in patients with this form of total hip replacement.

After 40-plus years of multiple investigations, creative problem solving, advances in molecular biology, innovative production of a perfected hip simulator, effective unraveling of a unique wear mechanism, and the deployment of a crosslinked polyethylene polymer, had we finally succeeded in preventing this mysterious bone destruction?

Again, the answer is a resounding *yes!*

In answering this question, the two most salient measures are (1) the incidence of cases of bone destruction and, perhaps even more important from the patient's point of view, (2) the number of patients forced to have a reoperation because of bone destruction and its consequences.

In detecting bone destruction in total hip replacements, x-rays have long been the universal standard. Large x-ray studies verified there was virtually no bone destruction in patients receiving our highly crosslinked polyethylene total hip replacements. Consider some of the evidence:

- Our study of 768 patients from six medical centers across North America found no bone destruction after 13 years.
- A study using the innovative larger femoral heads, which we made possible, showed no bone destruction after 10 years.
- A study of 74 of the most challenging patients—very young (average age, 41 years)—showed no bone destruction after 10 years. They had zero reoperations resulting from bone destruction and virtually no wear (on average, only 10 microns per year, or one 10th the thickness of a human hair per year).
- A review of 100 consecutive cases did find one case that appeared to have bone destruction after nine years, although the patient had no symptoms. Four years later, a follow-up x-ray showed no evidence of any progression of the bone destruction, leaving the original diagnosis in question in the absence of a biopsy.

These reports are illustrative of many others confirming either complete absence or very rare cases of bone destruction. Nearly all represent a large series of patients using crosslinked polyethylene for 10 years or more. In those unusual cases in which the x-rays suggested that bone destruction might exist, some degree of uncertainty remains, because none of these cases have been "biopsied"—meaning, none have been examined under the microscope. Even then, these cases are so uncommon that, if they were to be proved to be particle-induced bone destruction, they would most likely reflect the adage that they are the exceptions that prove the rule.

Because computed tomography (CT) has a much higher resolution than a standard x-ray examination, it is better able to detect very small areas of bone destruction. However, CT is expensive. It is never used routinely to evaluate total hip patients because it exposes them to greater x radiation and because the detection of very small lesions of bone destruction would not influence the care of the patient in any way. The small areas of bone destruction that could be found by CT but would not yet show up on x-rays would not cause pain, would not cause fractures, and would not loosen the prosthesis. If, over time, they were to enlarge enough to cause these problems, they would then be detectable by an x-ray.

One such small research study that used CT to examine young patients after a total hip replacement is illustrative. As noted before, young patients (younger than 50) with total hip replacements have the highest risk of wear because they are by far the most active, and, with conventional polyethylene, these young patients had the highest rate of bone destruction.

In this small research study, at six years after surgery, bone destruction was detected by CT at a rate of 24% in patients with conventional polyethylene and in just one instance (2%) among those with crosslinked polyethylene. Again, the one instance of purported bone destruction remains unproven because it was not examined under a microscope. Because there was no reason to do a biopsy, none was done.

Conceptually, we would have wished to explore that matter further to find out exactly what the nature of that situation was in this one patient, because we have a vested interest in the effects of the material. But the patient was completely symptom free and the area in question was very small; it had caused no trouble and was unlikely to cause any trouble for many years, if ever. So, although it is registered as a case of bone destruction, there is incomplete proof and, to date, no impact on the patient.

When studied using RSA, 12 patients who had our crosslinked polyethylene, six with a 28-millimeter femoral head size and six with a 36-millimeter head size, showed that after 13 years, the wear rates were very low; the rates remained the same during the entire time and they were the same for each head size. Head size made no difference in wear rate. Moreover, on the more sensitive CT examinations done in this research study, none showed bone destruction.

These findings of the study using CT, plus the RSA study, reinforce another report of 69 patients with 36-millimeter femoral heads or larger, moving against our crosslinked polyethylene for 11 years, again showing low wear, no increase in wear over time, and no bone destruction. In another report, even among patients with the greatest risk of wear, those young, active patients younger than 51 years of age, there was low wear, no change in wear over time, and no bone destruction.

The second, and perhaps even more critical measure of determining whether we had reduced bone destruction, is the number of patients who required a reoperation necessitated by bone destruction. In the future, such a study of the number of reoperations caused by *bone destruction alone* may become possible. At this time, in early 2017, the records automatically combine reoperations caused by bone destruction with those caused by *loosening* of components. Although this is a disadvantage, it is still well worth looking at the data.

The best information in the world on these reoperations comes from Australia, where the Australian National Joint Replacement Registry thoroughly surveys all total joint replacements throughout Australia. Among those with crosslinked polyethylene that required a reoperation for "loosening or bone destruction" after 10 years' use, the records show that the combined number of reoperations done for both reasons was astonishingly low: 1.1%!

When the Australian Registry followed up with these patients after three additional years, the result was exactly the same: 1.1%. This means that, even after 13 years, virtually 99% of the patients did not require a reoperation for *either* a loose component or bone destruction. Because of the high likelihood that at least some of these patients were reoperated for a prosthesis that had become loose without bone destruction, the actual number of patients reoperated on solely for bone destruction was almost certainly less than 1%. Moreover, after 13 years among patients using crosslinked polyethylene, revision operations for *any cause whatsoever* had been cut in half!

Similarly, in a massive study of more than 25,000 patients in California, crosslinked polyethylene cut the overall reoperation rate in half after only three to eight years.

This is a dramatic reduction in bone destruction! It is also a dramatic reduction in all reoperations. And also specifically for those done for bone destruction compared with the previous 40 years of use of the old polyethylene, for which reoperation rates for bone destruction reached 10% to 40%. In younger, more active patients, the occurrence of reoperations for bone destruction from conventional polyethylene in one type of cementless implant was 56%! These patients were all forced to undergo the complex, dangerous, and distinctly less satisfactory reoperations specifically because of the bone destruction from the old polyethylene.

Moreover, our prediction, based solely on our unanticipated hip simulator findings that it should be acceptable to use larger femoral heads because of the marked reduction of wear from the crosslinking, has been confirmed in patients by results with durations of 10 years and longer. Concomitantly and importantly, the ability of larger femoral heads to decrease the risk of dislocation strikingly for both primary total hip arthroplasty operations and for reoperations has been documented already in a large, prospective randomized controlled study, the strongest type of scientific study design. This is a totally unanticipated yet wonderful additional benefit of our commitment to the development of crosslinked polyethylene.

It is now widely recognized that crosslinked polyethylene in total hip replacements virtually eliminates both wear and bone destruction. This has resulted in a huge reduction of reoperations following total hip replacements worldwide.

Today, more than 90% of all total hip operations in the United States use crosslinked polyethylene. In fact, the nationwide report of the American Joint Replacement Registry of 2016 found that "surgeons in our sample overwhelmingly chose to use crosslinked polyethylene." The startling figures show that among 139,317 total hip replacement operations reported during 2012 through 2015, more than 98% used crosslinked polyethylene throughout each of these four years. This figure is truly remarkable.

Moreover, our work identifying that the crosslinking of the polyethylene was so highly wear resistant that it made possible the use of larger femoral balls than any used during the prior

40 years has resulted in an extraordinary change in the choice of head sizing. Larger heads (36 millimeters in diameter) were applied in *half* of all cases. Again, this is also truly remarkable.

Around the world, an estimated six million people are walking on total hip replacements using crosslinked polyethylene. This truly represents the conquest of a worldwide, totally unique disease, never seen before throughout human history.

Chapter 17

Reprise: The Reward of
the Clinician–Scientist

*The beginning of knowledge is
the discovery of something we do not understand.*
—FRANK HERBERT

Mark Bolger had a passion for skiing beyond anything else. His earliest memories were of a long, white, enticing slope of fresh powder in Aspen. Avid skiers themselves, his parents had snuck in a weekend at the ski resort six weeks before he was due to be born.

As his mother, Roxanne, sat at the lodge, watching his father showcase his skills on the mountain, Mark started squirming. Soon the contractions kicked in. "You couldn't wait to get out there!" she liked to tell him. "I swear, if we hadn't gone to Aspen, you'd never have been born early." Regardless of whether she was right, Mark always considered himself a native of the slopes and went skiing every chance he got.

One year, when he was skiing at one of his favorite resorts in New England, the ski lift broke. Mark fell 40 feet to the ground and broke his leg. The fracture occurred at the narrow part of the femur just below the ball (often referred to as the *femoral neck*).

The extreme force of the fall increased the risk of failure of repair of this fracture, because such violence tends to impair the blood supply. The prognosis was somewhat guarded. Because Mark was only 49 years old, and he had youth and fitness on his side, we expected his fracture to heal, but the blood supply to the ball of the femur is always a worry in these cases.

Three years later, Mark came back to see us. The blood supply had never fully recovered and his femoral ball had collapsed. When that happens, because the surface of the ball is no longer smooth, the cartilage in the socket also gets damaged.

I told Mark he would need a total hip replacement.

At this time (it was 1984), conventional polyethylene and cementless total hips were being used in hip implants. By the time Mark needed a total hip replacement, we had designed our cementless total hip replacement and felt it was ideal for such a relatively young man.

What we didn't know at the time was that the bone destruction we were seeing was not just cement disease, as everyone assumed. We wouldn't find out until later that other particles, those of the conventional polyethylene, were also involved.

Nonetheless, the operation and rehabilitation all went beautifully. Mark made a full recovery and went back to skiing happily for the next 17 years. By the time he had trouble with his hip again, so much time had passed that he had partially forgotten the accident and the operation!

Fortunately, our knowledge had progressed a lot during that interval. When Mark came to see me about pain from a 17-year-old hip implant using the old polyethylene, I was not at all surprised that his x-rays revealed extensive bone destruction, as well as loosening of the thigh piece.

Although this was early in our experience with our new crosslinked polyethylene, the experimental data were so strong and the disadvantage of putting conventional polyethylene back in was so obvious that we used our crosslinked polyethylene.

Among the many improvements in implant design that I had made in total hip surgery over the years, a very important one was the replaceable hip socket. Although the *replaceable socket design* that I invented in 1971 was initially for use with bone cement fixation to the skeleton, by 1984, I had advanced it to a cement-less design. This replaceable, or so-called *modular*, socket design meant that if a reoperation was needed and the outer metal shell was still well fixed to the pelvis, it would not have to be replaced. Only the plastic liner needed to be changed, markedly reducing the duration and the trauma of reoperation. This concept revolutionized socket reconstructions for both primary and for revision total hip operations, even in cases with very severe compromise of the bone from bone destruction. Almost all hip sockets used today follow this important innovation.

So I was able to give Mark the best available combination, highly crosslinked polyethylene inserted into a modular cement-less socket, despite the fact that the bone of his hip socket had been partially damaged by the bone destruction from his particle disease. The only remaining question was: How would the new polyethylene wear? That's where Mark Bolger becomes a stellar example.

At his 15-year follow-up examination from *that* operation, I compared his new x-rays with his early postoperative films. The results were thrilling. I could not identify any wear that had taken place. And, even more important, no bone destruction had occurred.

During that interview he asked the same question that Peter Dunn had asked years before, about my being both a clinician and an investigator. Again I replied affirmatively, using the term *clinician–scientist*. I said that the term described the juxtaposition of two critical but very diverse features of contemporary medicine.

"But," he countered, what does that phrase actually mean?"

It represents a fascinating but rapidly declining combination of two entirely separate key activities in medicine. Clinician–scientists are quickly becoming an "endangered species." They are those doctors who are clinicians *and* do research. These two activities have remarkably different intellectual and human characteristics. The reason for a decline in this category of physician is that it is clearly more efficient for any one practitioner of medical activities to be singularly focused on either one or the other.

Consider the differences in what each one does. In patient care, the guiding dictum requires that you do things you know will work well. Physicians must apply preferentially those therapies that have been shown to work. Patient care is not an experimental opportunity. The practice of medicine is and must be conservative. Yes, there clearly needs to be innovation in medicine, but it is almost exclusively limited to that small percentage of physicians who practice in an academic institution, and even there, most care must be those therapies that are known to work.

Clinical practice is also a deeply human interaction, requiring excellent interpersonal skills, the ability to instill confidence in patients regarding their care, along with compassion and empathy. For most medical interactions with most patients, innovation is not required.

Speaking specifically of the surgical care of patients, its central feature could be described as "crisis management." Society allows surgeons to do things in the operating room for which they would be arrested if they did the same thing out on the street. The reason that surgeons are permitted to take a knife and incise a patient's body is because of the overriding dictum that, to the fullest extent possible, this can only be permitted when it is in the very best interests of the patient.

In addition, surgery has another very special aspect. There is no instant replay. The demands of surgery are such that it is something that is done *now*, done under stress, and it does not encourage delay, procrastination, or indecision.

Contrast those features with the science of improving the management of disease. This aspect of medical endeavors is not conservative. In fact, if medical scientists only do what has already been proved to work well, they are abject failures. Innovation is *required*.

In contrast with performing surgery, doing research does not require a daily exercise in "crisis management." Also, the time horizon is entirely different. In the clinical practice of medicine, the results of care are often relatively rapid and are generally well-known fairly quickly. In research, ideas may take years or decades to develop. Equally so, in research there is, of necessity, a high percentage of failure. Nor is there is a major requirement for the personal qualities of empathy, compassion, or the ability to instill confidence in a patient. Thus, the two activities are remarkably dissimilar, although united by a common desire for optimizing the outcome for patients.

Another important difference is that patient care is generally given one person at a time. Conversely, if success is achieved in the laboratory, it is possible to influence the care of millions of patients, patients many miles away, and for decades into the future.

For Mark and for so many others, our research had worked brilliantly. This outcome is the truest reward for the clinician's contract.

Our 40-plus-year quest had been challenging, fascinating, daunting, intriguing, and richly rewarding. All patients who require a total hip operation today—and forever into the future—do so with a vastly greater probability of long-term success.

The conquest of particle-induced bone destruction has also been remarkable because our first startling observation of massive bone destruction around the prosthesis of a total hip replacement was an example of a disease that had never existed before in all of human history. The sheets of macrophages associated with aggressive bone destruction were a surprise to everyone.

After that discovery, the pathway to a solution to this problem was nothing less than torturous. At its peak, this unique new disease affected more than one million people around the world. Among certain patient groups, 40% to 60% suffered from the disease, especially younger, more active patients. Reoperation rates reached 10% to 40%, depending on the prosthesis and patient profile.

Hans Willert's recognition that particles of bone cement could activate macrophages was absolutely critical and led to the designation *cement disease*. For many years, it was assumed that activation was caused *only* by bone cement. As a result, there was a massive shift to cementless prostheses. But that shift led, once again, to dismay.

When we realized bone destruction occurred in the complete absence of bone cement, we identified the cause more accurately as *particle disease* instead. The dominating particle was the tiny wear particle from wear of the polyethylene. Because of its near-constant motion at the hip joint, the total hip replacement had inadvertently proved to be an internal, highly efficient *particle generator!*

The inability of the macrophages to destroy either the particles of polyethylene or bone cement had ultimately led to the stimulation of osteoclasts, which destroyed the bone. This led to a major shift away from conventional polyethylene to the three alternate bearings: metal on metal, ceramic on ceramic and metal on crosslinked polyethylene.

Metal-on-metal implants had long been known to produce enormous quantities of metal debris particles, but no serious consequences had been previously reported. After the turn of this century, the number of metal-on-metal implants increased in the United States to approximately 40% of all total hip replacements. It was only then that the reports of uniquely serious complications emerged and took a heavy toll. For many patients, metal-on-metal implants proved devastating.

Despite all these severe failures, the magnificence of total hip replacement and its remarkable successes compelled researchers to attack this strange particle disease. Our decision to attempt to solve the bone destruction problem led us on a circuitous adventure. We encountered an unexpected need to create a precisely accurate hip simulator. To do this, we needed to understand the human gait at a level never before appreciated.

Thanks to the many patients who bequeathed us their total hip implants, we were able to make the critical observations that led to our unique hypothesis: If we stop the reorientation of the polymer molecule caused by the forces of gait, we will block the generation of wear particles.

My alliance with Ed Merrill and Orhun Muratoglu from MIT began our complex development of crosslinked polyethylene. After fires, explosions, bomb scares, lawsuits, and bankruptcies, our crosslinked polyethylene finally made it to market.

Now, 18 years after its first use, we have overwhelming proof that crosslinking drastically reduces both wear and bone destruction in patients. Our concerns about complications from the use of our crosslinked polyethylene resulting from issues of oxidation and issues of decreased fatigue strength proved to be unrealized.

A lifetime of the combination of clinical practice and research yielded us a most magnificent reward: the conquest of a worldwide disease!

APPENDIX A

Further Reading

CHAPTER 1: THE GAME IS AFOOT!

Harris WH, Schiller AL, Scholler J-M, Freiberg RA, Scott R. Extensive localized bone reabsorption in the femur following total hip replacement. *J Bone Joint Surg.* 1976; 58-A(5): 612–618.

CHAPTER 2: THE CART BEFORE THE HORSE

Charnley J. *Low Friction Arthroplasty of the Hip: Theory and Practice.* New York, NY: Springer-Verlag, 1979.

CHAPTER 3: UNIQUELY CREATIVE, BUT DANGEROUS

Maradit Kremers H, Larson DR, Crowson CS, et al. Prevalence of total hip (THA) and total knee (TKA) arthroplasty in the United States. Presented at the Academy of Orthopaedic Surgeons annual meeting; New Orleans, Louisiana; March 11–14, 2014.

Mayo Clinic. Clinical updates: First nationwide prevalence study of hip and knee arthroplasty shows 7.2 million Americans living with implants. 2014. http://www.mayoclinic.org/medical-professionals/clinical-updates/orthopaedic-surgery/study-hip-knee-arthroplasty-shows-7-2-million-americans-living-with-implants.

CHAPTER 4: THE FIRST REAL BREAKTHROUGH

DeLee J, Charnley J. Radiological demarcation of cemented sockets in total hip replacement. *Clin Orthop Rel Res.* 1976; 121: 20–32.

Willert HG. Reactions of the articular capsule to wear products of artificial joint prostheses. *J Biomed Mater Res.* 1977; 11(2): 157–164.

Jones LC, Hungerford DS. Cement disease. *Clin Orthop Rel Res.* 1987; 225: 192–206.

Maloney WJ, Jasty M, Harris WH, Galante JO, Callaghan JJ. Endosteal erosion in association with stable uncemented femoral components. *J Bone Joint Surg.* 1990; 72-A(7): 1025–1034.

Mulroy RD Jr, Mankin HJ, Harris WH. Insertion of a prosthetic hip into a total hip allograft. *J. Bone Joint Surg.* 1990; 72-B(4): 643–646.

Schmalzried TP, Jasty M, Harris WH. Periprosthetic bone loss in total hip arthroplasty. *J Bone Joint Surg.* 1992; 74-A: 849–863.

Schmalzried TP, Kwong LM, Jasty M, et al. The mechanism of loosening of cemented acetabular components in total hip arthroplasty. *Clin Orthop Rel Res.* 1992; 274: 60–78.

Bobyn JD, Jacobs JJ, Tanzer M, et al. The susceptibility of smooth implant surfaces to periimplant fibrosis and migration of polyethylene wear debris. *Clin Orthop Rel Res.* 1995; 311: 21–39.

Harris WH. The problem is osteolysis. *Clin Orthop Rel Res.* 1995; 311: 46–53.

Zicat B, Engh CA, Gokcen E. Patterns of osteolysis around total hip components inserted with and without cement. *J Bone Joint Surg.* 1995; 777-A(3): 432–439.

Perez RE, Rodriguez JA, Deshmukh RG, Ranawat CS. Polyethylene wear and periprosthetic osteolysis in metal-backed acetabular components with cylindrical liners. *J Arthroplasty.* 1996; 13(1): 1–7.

Dorr LD, Lewonowski K, Lucero M, Harris M, Wan Z. Failure mechanisms of anatomic porous replacement in cementless total hip replacement. *Clin Orthop Rel Res.* 1997; 334: 157–167.

Clohisy JC, Harris WH. The Harris–Galante uncemented femoral component in primary total hip replacement at 10 years. *J Arthroplasty.* 1999; 14(8): 915–917.

Hellman EJ, Capello WN, Feinberg JR. Omnifit cementless total hip arthroplasty. *Clin Orthop Rel Res.* 1999; 364: 164–174.

Claus AM, Sychterz CJ, Hopper RH Jr, Engh CA. Pattern of osteolysis around two different cementless metal-backed cups. *J Arthroplasty.* 2001; 16(8), Suppl 1: 177–182.

Duffy GP, Berry DJ, Rowland C, Cabanela ME. Primary uncemented total hip arthroplasty in patients <40 years old. *J Arthroplasty*. 2001; 16(8), Suppl 1: 140–144.

Harris WH. Wear and periprosthetic osteolysis: The problem. *Clin Orthop Rel Res*. 2001; 393: 66–70.

Crowther JD, Lachiewicz PF. Survival and polyethylene wear of porous-coated acetabular components in patients less than fifty years old. *J Bone Joint Surg*. 2002; 84(5): 729–735.

Harris WH. Results of uncemented cups: A critical appraisal at 15 years. *Clin Orthop Rel Res*. 2003; 417: 121–125.

Duffy P, Sher JL, Partington PF. Premature wear and osteolysis in an HA-coated, uncemented total hip arthroplasty. *J Bone Joint Surg*. 2004; 86-B(1): 34–38.

Sanchez-Sotelo J, Lewallen DG, Harmsen WS, Harrington J, Cabanela ME. Comparison of wear and osteolysis in hip replacement using two different coatings of the femoral stem. *Int Orthop*. 2004; 28: 206–210.

Hallan G, Lie SA, Havelin LI. High wear rates and extensive osteolysis in 3 types of uncemented total hip arthroplasty. *Acta Orthop*. 2006; 77(4): 575–584.

CHAPTER 5: MEANWHILE, BACK AT THE RANCH...

Charnley J, Feagin JA. Low friction arthroplasty in congenital subluxation of the hip. *Clin Orthop Rel Res*. 1973; March–April(91): 98–113.

Harris WH. Total hip replacement for congenital dysplasia of the hip: Technique. In: Harris WH, ed. *The Hip: Proceedings of the Second Open Scientific Session of the Hip Society*. St. Louis, MO: C.V. Mosby; 1974: 251–265.

Harris WH, Crothers OD. Autogenous bone grafting using the femoral head to correct severe acetabular deficiency for total hip replacement. In: Evarts CM, ed. *The Hip: Proceedings of the Fourth Open Scientific Meeting*. St. Louis, MO: C.V. Mosby; 1976: 161–185.

Harris WH, Crothers O, Oh I. Total hip replacement and femoral-head bone-grafting for severe acetabular deficiency in adults. *J Bone Joint Surg*. 1977; 59-A: 752–759.

Harris, WH. Total hip replacement for osteoarthritis secondary to congenital dysplasia or congenital dislocation of the hip. *Int Orthop*. 1978; 2: 127–138.

Woolson ST, Harris WH. Complex total hip replacement for dysplastic or hypoplastic hips using miniature or microminiature components. *J Bone Joint Surg.* 1983; 65-A: 1099–1108.

Harris WH. Bone grafting for acetabular deficiency in association with total replacement. In: Brand RA, ed. *The Hip: Proceedings of the Fourteenth Open Scientific Meeting of the Hip Society.* St. Louis, MO: C.V. Mosby; 1986: 94–119.

Jasty M, Harris WH. Total hip reconstruction using frozen femoral head allografts in patients with acetabular bone loss. *Orthop Clin North Am.* 1987; 18: 291–299.

Mulroy RD Jr, Harris WH. Failure of acetabular autogenous grafts in total hip arthroplasty: Increasing incidence: A follow-up note. *J Bone Joint Surg.* 1990; 72-A: 1536–1540.

Kwong LM, Jasty M, Harris WH. High failure rate of bulk femoral head allografts in total hip acetabular reconstructions at 10 years. *J Arthroplasty.* 1993; 8: 341–346.

Jasty M, Anderson MJ, Harris WH. Total hip replacement for developmental dysplasia of the hip. *Clin Orthop.* 1995; 311: 40–45.

Harris, WH. Total hip arthroplasty in the management of congenital hip dislocation. In: Callaghan JJ, Rosenberg AG, Rubash HE, eds. *The Adult Hip.* Philadelphia, PA: Lippincott-Raven Publishers; 1998: 1165–1182.

Dearborn JT, Harris WH. Acetabular revision after failed total hip arthroplasty in patients with congenital hip dislocation and dysplasia: Results after a mean of 8.6 years. *J Bone Joint Surg.* 2000; 82-A(8): 1146–1153.

CHAPTER 6: IS IT REALLY CEMENT DISEASE?

Willert HG, Semlitsch M. Reactions of the articular joint capsule to wear products of artificial joint prostheses. *J Biomed Mater Res.* 1977; 11: 157–164.

Goldring SR, Schiller AL, Roelke M, Rourke CM, O'Neill DA, Harris WH. The synovial-like membrane at the bone–cement interface in loose total hip replacements and its proposed role in bone lysis. *J Bone Joint Surg.* 1983; 65-A: 575–583.

Willert HG, Bertram H, Buchhorn GH. Osteolysis in alloarthroplasty of the hip. *Clin Orthop Rel Res.* 1990; 258: 108–120.

Kwong LM, Jasty M, Mulroy RD, Maloney WJ, Bragdon CR, Harris WH. The histology of the radiolucent line. *J Bone Joint Surg.* 1992; 74-B: 67–73.

Schmalzried TP, Kwong LM, Jasty M, et al. The mechanism of loosening of cemented acetabular components in total hip arthroplasty. *Clin Orthop Rel Res.* 1992; 274: 60–78.

Schmalzried TP, Jasty M, Harris WH. Periprosthetic bone loss in total hip arthroplasty. *J Bone Joint Surg.* 1992; 74-A: 849–863.

Jiranek WA, Michado M, Jasty M, et al. Production of cytokines around loosened cemented acetabular components. *J Bone Joint Surg.* 1993; 75-A(6): 863–879.

Kabo JM, Gebhard JS, Loren G, Amstutz HC. In vivo wear of polyethylene acetabular components. *J Bone Joint Surg.* 1993; 75-B: 254–258.

Jasty M, Bragdon CR, Jiranek W, Chandler H, Maloney W, Harris WH. Etiology of osteolysis around porous-coated cementless total hip arthroplasties. *Clin Orthop Rel Res.* 1994; 308: 111–126.

Willert HG, Semlitsch M. Tissue reactions to plastic and metallic wear products of joint endoprostheses. *Clin Orthop Rel Res.* 1996; 333: 4–14.

Shanbhag AS, Hasselman CT, Rubash HE. The John Charnley Award: Inhibition of wear debris mediated osteolysis in a canine total hip arthroplasty model. *Clin Orthop Rel Res.* 1997; November(344): 33–43.

Jacobs JJ, Roebuck KA, Archibeck M, Hallab NJ, Glant TT. Osteolysis: Basic science. *Clin Orthop Rel Res.* 2001; December(393): 71–77.

Archibeck M J, Jacobs JJ, Roebuck KA, Glant TT. The basic science of periprosthetic osteolysis. *Instr Course Lect.* 2001; 50: 185–195.

Goodman SB, Gibon E, Yao Z. The basic science of periprosthetic osteolysis. *PMC Instr Course Lect.* 2013; 62: 201–206.

CHAPTER 7: AN UNEXPECTED FIRST STEP

McKee GK, Watson-Farrar J. Replacement of arthritic hips by the Mckee–Farrar prosthesis. *J Bone Joint Surg.* 1966; 48-B(2): 245–258.

Boutin P. Total arthroplasty of the hip with aluminum prostheses. *Acta Orthop Belg.* 1974; 40(5–6): 744–754. [In French].

Wright TM, Fukubashi T, Burstein AH. The effect of carbon fiber reinforcement on contact area, contact pressure, and time-dependent deformation in polyethylene tibial components. *J Biomed Mater Res.* 1981; 15(5): 719–730.

Mintz L, Tsao AK, McCrae CR, Stulberg SD, Wright T. The arthroscopic evaluation and characteristics of severe polyethylene wear in total knee arthroplasty. *Clin Orthop Rel Res.* 1991; 273: 215–222.

Schmalzried TP, Jasty M, Harris WH. Periprosthetic bone loss in total hip arthroplasty: Polyethylene wear debris and the concept of the effective joint space. *J Bone Joint Surg.* 1992; 74-A: 849–863.

Tanzer M, Maloney WJ, Jasty M, Harris WH. The progression of femoral cortical osteolysis in association with total hip arthroplasty without cement. *J Bone Joint Surg.* 1992; 74-A(3): 404–410.

Li S, Burstein AH. Ultra-high molecular weight polyethylene. *J Bone Joint Surg.* 1994; 76-A: 1080–1090.

Harris WH. The problem is osteolysis. *Clin Orthop Rel Res.* 1995; 311: 46–53.

Smith E, Harris WH. Increasing prevalence of femoral lysis in cementless total hip arthroplasty. *J Arthroplasty.* 1995; 10: 407–412.

Bragdon CR, O'Connor DO, Lowenstein JD, Jasty M, Syniuta WD. The importance of multidirectional motion on the wear of polyethylene. *Proc Inst Mech Eng (H).* 1996; 210(3): 157–165.

Chmell MJ, Poss R, Thomas WH, Sledge CB. Early failure of Hylamer acetabular inserts due to eccentric wear. *J Arthroplasty.* 1996; 11(3): 351–353.

Ramamurti BS, Bragdon CR, O'Connor DO, et al. Loci of movement of selected points on the femoral head during normal gait: Three-dimensional computer simulation. *J Arthroplasty.* 1996; 11: 845–852.

Livingston BJ, Chmell MJ, Spector M, Poss R. Complications of total hip arthroplasty associated with the use of an acetabular component with a Hylamer liner. *J Bone Joint Surg.* 1997; 79-A: 1529–1538.

Sychterz CJ, Young AM, McAuley JP, Engh CA. Comparison of head penetration into Hylamer and Enduron polyethylene liners. *J Arthroplasty.* 2000; 15(3): 372–374.

Harris WH. Wear and periprosthetic osteolysis: The problem. *Clin Orthop Rel Res.* 2001; 393: 66–70.

Dumbleton JH, Manley MT, Edidin AA. A literature review of the association between wear rate and osteolysis in total hip arthroplasty. *J Arthroplasty.* 2002; 17: 649–661.

Willert HG, Buckhorn GH, Fayyazi A, Flury R, Windler M, Lohmann CH. Metal-on-metal bearings and hypersensitivity in patients with artificial hip joints: A clinical and histomorphological study. *J Bone Joint Surg.* 2005; 87(1): 28–36.

Malchau H, Bragdon CR, Muratoglu OK. The stepwise introduction of innovation into orthopaedic surgery: The next level of dilemmas. *J Arthroplasty.* 2011 September(26): 825–831.

CHAPTER 8: FLYING BLIND

Charnley J. Anchorage of the femoral head prosthesis to the shaft of the femur. *J Bone Joint Surg.* 1960; 42-B: 28–30.

Schmalzreid TP, Peters PC, Maurer BT, Bragdon CR, Harris WH. Long-duration metal-on-metal total hip arthroplasties with low wear of the articulating surfaces. *J Arthroplasty.* 1996; 11: 322–331.

Jasty M, Goetz DD, Bragdon CR, et al. Wear of polyethylene acetabular components in total hip arthroplasty: An analysis of 128 components retrieved at autopsy or revision operations. *J Bone Joint Surg.* 1997; 79-A: 349–358.

Bomex PF, Morcuende J. A historical and economic perspective on Sir John Charnley, Chas F. Thackray Limited, and the early arthroplasty industry. *Iowa Orthop J.* 2005; 25: 30–37.

van Hilten, LG. Why it's time to publish research "failures." Elsevier. May 5, 2015. http://www.elsevier.com/connect/scientists-we-want-your-negative-results-too.

CHAPTER 9: THE GAMBLE PAYS OFF

Newton, I, as cited in Edwards, T. *A Dictionary of Thoughts: Being a Cyclopedia of Laconic Quotations from the Best Authors, Both Ancient and Modern.* London, Cassell Publishing, 1891, p. 120. https://books.google.com/books?id=zGY9AAAAYAAJ&vq=Isaac+Newton&dq=If+I+have+ever+made+any+valuable+discoveries,+Newton+source&source=gbs_navlinks_s.

Hosler D, Burkett SL, Tarkanian, MJ. Prehistoric polymers: Rubber processing in ancient Mesoamerica. *Science.* 1999; 284(5422): 1988–1991.

Geselowitz M. Oral history: Edward Merrill. IEEE History Center, The Institute of Electrical and Electronics Engineering, Inc. February 22, 2001. http://ethw.org/Oral-History:Edward_Merrill.

Dwyer D. Mass General Hospital ranked best hospital in the land. Boston.com. July 21, 2015. http://www.boston.com/health/2015/07/21/mgh-ranked-best-hospital-the-land/Ubq2dxTNqSRn1zshQmgqSJ/story.html.

CHAPTER 10: SUCCESS AT LAST!

Jasty M, Goetz DD, Bragdon CR, et al. Wear of polyethylene acetabular components in total hip arthroplasty. *J Bone Joint Surg.* 1997; 79-A(3): 349–358.

McKellop H, Shen F, Lu B, Campbell P, Salovey R. Development of an extremely wear-resistant ultra high molecular weight polyethylene for total hip replacements. *J Orthop Res.* 1999; 17: 157–167.

Muratoglu OK, Bragdon CR, O'Connor D, et al. Larger diameter femoral heads used in conjunction with a highly crosslinked ultra-high molecular weight polyethylene: A new concept. *J Arthroplasty.* 2001; 16(8), Suppl 1: 24–30.

Muratoglu OK, Harris WH. Use of highly crosslinked ultra-high molecular weight polyethylene in total hip replacement to decrease the generation of wear debris and reduce periprosthetic osteolysis. *Semin Arthroplasty.* 2002; 13(4): 318–324.

Bragdon CR, Jasty M, Muratoglu OK, O'Connor DO, Harris WH. Third-body wear of highly crosslinked polyethylene in a hip simulator. *J Arthroplasty.* 2003; 18(5): 553–561.

Bragdon CR, Jasty M, Muratoglu OK, Harris WH. Third-body wear testing of a highly crosslinked acetabular liner: The effect of large femoral head size in the presence of particulate poly(methyl-methacrylate) debris. *J Arthroplasty.* 2005; 20(3): 379–385.

Wannomae KK, Christensen SD, Freiberg AA, Bhattacharyya S, Harris WH, Muratoglu OK. The effect of real-time aging on the oxidation and wear of highly crosslinked UHMWPE acetabular liners. *Biomaterials.* 2006; 27(9): 1980–1987.

Estok DM II, Burroughs BR, Muratoglu OK, Harris WH. Comparison of hip simulator wear of 2 different highly crosslinked ultra high molecular weight polyethylene acetabular components using both 32- and 38-mm femoral heads. *J Arthroplasty.* 2007; 22(4): 581–589.

Plank GR, Estok DM II, Muratoglu OK, O'Connor DO, Burroughs BR, Harris WH. Contact stress assessment of conventional and highly crosslinked ultra high molecular weight polyethylene acetabular liners with finite element analysis and pressure sensitive film. *J Biomed Mater Res.* 2007; 80(1): 1–10.

Laurent MP, Johnson TS, Crowninshield RD, Blanchard CR, Bhambri SK, Yao JQ. Characterization of a highly crosslinked ultrahigh molecular weight polyethylene in clinical use in total hip arthroplasty. *J Arthroplasty.* 2008; 23(5): 751–761.

Anseth S, Pulido PA, Adelson WS, Patil SP, Sandwell JC, Colwell CW Jr. Fifteen-year to twenty-year results of cementless Harris–Galante porous femoral and Harris–Galante porous I and II acetabular components. *J Arthroplasty.* 2010; 45(5): 687–691.

Milner GR, Boldsen JL. Humeral and femoral head diameters in recent white American skeletons. *J Forensic Sci.* 2012; 57(1): 35–40.

Goel A, Lau EC, Ong KL, Berry DJ, Malkani AL. Dislocation rates following primary total hip arthroplasty have plateaued in the Medicare population. *J Arthroplasty.* 2015; 30: 743–746.

CHAPTER 11: TERRA INCOGNITA

Bloomberg Business. Are patent problems stifling U.S. innovation? April 8, 2009. http://www.bloomberg.com/bw/stories/2009-04-08/are-patent-problems-stifling-u-dot-s-dot-innovation-businessweek-business-news-stock-market- and-financial-advice.

Pellegrino News. Most valuable patent in history expires. July 25, 2011. http://www.pellegrinoandassociates.com/most-valuable-patent-in-history-expires/.

Brachmann S. Top 10 patents for 2014. IPWatch. December 30, 2014. http://www.ipwatchdog.com/2014/12/30/52944/id=52944/.

U.S. Food and Drug Administration. About the FDA. March 23, 2015. http://www.fda.gov/AboutFDA/WhatWeDo/History/.

CNBC. Weird or genius? September 2, 2015. http://www.cnbc.com/2015/09/02/weird-or-genius-check-out-these-5-patents-from-the-past.html.

CHAPTER 12: SUDDENLY, TO THE FDA

duPlessis TA, Grobbelaar CJ, Marias F. The improvement of polyethylene prostheses through radiation crosslinking. *Radiat Phys Chem.* 1977; 9: 647–652.

Grobbelaar CJ, Plessis TAD, Marais F. The radiation improvement of polyethylene prostheses. *J Bone Joint Surg Br.* 1978; 60: 370–374.

Oonishi H, Takayama Y, Tsuji E. Improvement of polyethylene by irradiation in artificial joints. *Radiat Phys Chem.* 1992; 39: 495.

Oonishi H. Long-term clinical results of THR: Clinical results of THR of an alumina head with a crosslinked UHMWPE cup. *Orthop Surg Traumatol.* 1995; 38: 1255.

Wrobleski BM, Siney PD, Dowson D, Colling SN. Prospective clinical and joint simulator studies of a new total hip arthroplasty using alumina ceramic heads and crosslinked polyethylene cups. *J Bone Joint Surg Br.* 1996; 78: 280.

Grobbelaar CJ, Weber FA, Spirakis D, DuPlessis TA, Cappert G, Cakie JN. Clinical experience with gamma irradiation-crosslinked polyethylene: A 14 to 20 year follow up report. *South Afr Bone Joint Surg.* 1999; 11: 140.

Wroblewski B, Siney P, Fleming P. Low-friction arthroplasty of the hip using alumina ceramic and crosslinked polyethylene: A ten-year follow-up report. *J Bone Joint Surg Br.* 1999; 81: 54–55.

CHAPTER 14: UNFORESEEN COMPLICATIONS

Thanner J, Fring-Larson C, Kanholm J, Malchau H, Wessler B. Evaluation of Boneloc chemical and mechanical properties and a randomized clinical study of 30 total hip arthroplasties. *Acta Orthop Scand.* 1995; 6: 207–214.

Karrholm J, Herberts P, Hultmark P, Malchau H, Neibrandt B, Thanner J. Radiostereometry of hip prostheses: Review of methodology and clinical results. *Clin Orthop Rel Res.* 1997; 344: 94–110.

Martell JM, Berkson E, Berger R, Jacobs J. Comparison of two and three-dimensional computerized polyethylene wear analysis after total hip arthroplasty. *J Bone Joint Surg Am.* 2003; 85-A(6): 1111–1117.

CHAPTER 15: PANIC

Muratoglu OK, Bragdon CR, O'Connor DO, Jasty M, Harris WH. A novel method of cross-linking ultra-high-molecular-weight polyethylene to improve wear, reduce oxidation, and retain mechanical properties. *J Arthroplasty.* 2001; 16(2): 149–160.

Muratoglu OK, Ruberti J, Melotti S, Spiegelberg SH, Greenbaum ES, Harris WH. Optical analysis of surface changes on early retrievals of highly cross-linked and conventional polyethylene tibial inserts. *J Arthroplasty.* 2003; 18(7), Suppl 1: 42–47.

Muratoglu OK, Greenbaum ES, Bragdon CR, Jasty M, Freiberg AA, Harris WH. Surface analysis of early retrieved acetabular polyethylene liners: A comparison of conventional and highly cross-linked polyethylenes. *J Arthroplasty.* 2004; 19(1): 68–77.

Jasty M, Rubash H, Muratoglu OK. Highly cross-linked polyethylene: The debate is over—in the affirmative. *J Arthroplasty.* 2005; 20(4), Suppl 2: 55–58.

Langton DJ, Jameson SS, Joyce TJ, Hallab HJ, Natu S, Nargol AV. Early failure of metal-on-metal bearings in hip resurfacing and large diameter total hip replacement: A consequence of excess wear. *J Bone Joint Surg.* 2010; 92: 38–46.

Cohen D. Out of joint: The story of the ASR. *BMJ*. 2011; 342. [doi: http://dx.doi.org/10.1136/bmj.d2905].

Meier B. Metal hips failing fast, report says. *The New York Times*, Health Section. September 15, 2011, p. B1.

Meier B. Failure of artificial hip is expected to cost billions. *The Boston Globe*, Business Section. December 28, 2011, p. B9.

Meier B. FDA seeks to tighten regulations of all-metal hip implants. *The New York Times*. January 16, 2013, p. B1.

CHAPTER 16: UBIQUITOUS SUCCESS

Muratoglu OK, Bragdon CR, O'Connor DO, Jasty M, Harris WH. A novel method of crosslinking ultra-high molecular weight polyethylene to improve wear, reduce oxidation, and retain mechanical properties. Recipient of the HAP Paul Award. *J Arthroplasty*. 2001; 16(2): 149–160.

Digas G, Karrholm J, Thanner J, Malchau H, Herberts P. The Otto AuFranc Award: Highly cross-linked polyethylene in total hip arthroplasty: Randomized evaluation of penetration rate in cemented and uncemented sockets using radiostereometric analysis. *Clin Orthop Rel Res*. 2004; 429(6): 6–18.

Muratoglu OK, Greenbaum ES, Bragdon CR, Jasty M, Freiberg AA, Harris WH. Surface analysis of early retrieved acetabular polyethylene liners: A comparison of conventional and highly crosslinked polyethylenes. *J Arthroplasty*. 2004; 19(1): 68–77.

Geller JA, Malchau H, Bragdon C, Greene M, Harris WH, Freiberg AA. Large diameter femoral heads on highly cross-linked polyethylene: Minimum 3-year results. *Clin Orthop Rel Res*. 2006; 447: 53–59.

Bragdon CR, Greene M, Freiberg AA, Harris WH, Malchau H. Radiostereometric analysis comparison of wear of highly cross-linked polyethylene against 36- vs 28-mm femoral heads. *J Arthroplasty*. 2007; 22(6), Suppl 2: 125–129.

Geraint ER, Thomas GE, Simpson DJ, et al. The seven-year wear of highly cross-linked polyethylene in total hip arthroplasty: A double-blind, randomized controlled trial using radiostereometric analysis. *J Bone Joint Surg*. 2011; 93: 716–722.

Kurtz SM, Gawel HA, Patel JD. History and systematic review of wear and osteolysis outcomes for first-generation highly crosslinked polyethylene. *Clin Orthop Rel Res*. 2011; 469: 2262–2277.

Mall NA, Nunley RM, Zhu JJ, Maloney WJ, Barrack RL, Clohisy JC. The incidence of acetabular osteolysis in young patients with conventional versus highly crosslinked polyethylene. *Clin Orthop Rel Res.* 2011; 469(2): 372–381.

Engh CA Jr, Hopper RH Jr, Huynh C, Ho H, Sritulanondha S, Engh CA Sr. A prospective, randomized study of cross-linked and non-cross-linked polyethylene for total hip arthroplasty at 10-year follow-up. *J Arthroplasty.* 2012; 27(8): 2–8.

Garbuz DS, Masri BA, Duncan CP, et al. Do large heads (36 and 40 mm) result in reduced dislocation rates in a randomized clinical trial? *Clin Orthop Rel Res.* 2012; 470: 351–356.

Howie DW, Holubowycz OT, Middleton R, and the Large Articulation Study Group. Large femoral heads decrease the incidence of dislocation after total hip arthroplasty. *J Bone Joint Surg.* 2012; 94-A(12): 1095–1102.

Johanson P, Digas G, Herberts P. Highly crosslinked polyethylene does not reduce aseptic loosening in cemented THA: 10-Year findings of a randomized study. *Clin Orthop Rel Res.* 2012; 470(11): 3083–3093.

Yeung E, Bott PT, Chana R, et al. Mid-term results of third-generation alumina-on-alumina ceramic bearings in cementless total hip arthroplasty: A ten-year minimum follow-up. *J Bone Joint Surg.* 2012; 94-A(2): 138–144.

Babovic N, Trousdale, RT. Total hip arthroplasty using highly cross-linked polyethylene in patients younger than 50 years with minimum 10-year follow-up. *J Arthroplasty.* 2013; 28: 815–817.

Bragdon CR, Doerner M, Martell J, Jarrett B, Palm H, Multicenter Study Group, Malchau H. Clinical multicenter studies of the wear performance of highly crosslinked remelted polyethylene in THA. *Clin Orthop Rel Res.* 2013; 471: 393–402.

Bragdon C, Doerner M, Rubash H, et al. Clinical multi-centric studies of the wear performance of highly crosslinked remelted polyethylene in THR. *Clin Orthop Rel Res.* 2013; 471(2): 393–402.

Garcia-Rey R, Garcia-Cimbrelo E, Cruz-Pardos A. New polyethylenes in total hip replacement: A 10-to-12-year follow up study. *Bone Joint J.* 2013; 95: 326–332.

Kim Y-H, Park J-W, Patel C, Kim D-Y. Polyethylene wear and osteolysis after cementless total hip arthroplasty with alumina-on-highly crosslinked polyethylene bearings in patients younger than thirty years of age. *J Bone Joint Surg.* 2013; 95: 1088–1093.

Lachiewicz PF, Soileau ES. Low early and late dislocation rates with 36- and 40-mm heads in patients at high risk for dislocation. *Clin Orthop Rel Res.* 2013; 471(2): 439–443.

Australian Orthopaedic Association National Joint Replacement Registry. *Annual Report 2014: Hip and Knee Arthroplasty.* Adelaide: Australian Orthopaedic Association, 2014: 95.

Bedard NA, Callaghan JJ, Stefl MD, Willman TJ, Liu SS, Goetz DD. Fixation and wear with a contemporary acetabular component and cross-linked polyethylene at minimum 10-year follow-up. *J Arthroplasty.* 2014; 29: 1961–1969.

Callary SA, Solomon LB, Holubowycz OT, Campbell DG, Munn Z, Howie DW. Wear of highly crosslinked polyethylene acetabular components: A review of RSA studies. *Acta Orthop.* 2014; 86(2): 159–168.

Devane PA, Horne JG, Ashmore A, Mutimer J, Calvert G. A randomized prospective double-blind trial comparing X-linked with conventional polyethylene in THA: Minimum 10 year results. Presented at a closed meeting of the International Hip Society; Rio de Janeiro, Brazil; November 20–22, 2014.

Goel A, Lau EC, Ong KL, Berry DJ, Malkani AL. Dislocation rates following primary total hip arthroplasty have plateaued in the Medicare population. *J Arthroplasty.* 2015; 30(5): 743–746.

Snir N, Kaye ID, Klifto CS, et al. 10-Year follow-up wear analysis of first-generation highly crosslinked polyethylene in primary total hip arthroplasty. *J Arthroplasty.* 2014; 29: 630–633.

Bragdon CR, Barr CJ, Nielsen CS, et al. Minimum 10-year multi-center study of THR with highly cross-linked polyethylene and large diameter femoral heads. Presented at The Hip Society; Dallas, Texas; November 5–8, 2015.

Garvin KL, White TC, Dusad A, Hartman CW, Martell J. Low wear rates seen in THAs with highly crosslinked polyethylene at 9 to 14 years in patients younger than age 50 years. *Clin Orthop Rel Res.* 2015; 473: 3829–3835.

Glyn-Jones S, Geraint ERT, Garfield-Roberts P, et al. Highly crosslinked polyethylene in total hip arthroplasty decreases long-term wear: A double-blind randomized trial. *Clin Orthop Rel Res.* 2015; 473: 432–438.

Goodman SB. Editorial comment: 2014 Hip Society proceedings. *Clin Orthop Rel Res.* 2015; 473: 430–431.

Joyce TJ. Highly crosslinked polyethylene in total hip arthroplasty decreases long-term wear: A double-blind randomized trial. *Clin Orthop Rel Res.* 2015; 473: 439–440.

Lombardi AV, Berend KR, Morris MJ, Adams JB, Sneller MA. Large diameter metal-on- metal total hip arthroplasty: Dislocation infrequent but survivorship poor. *Clin Orthop Rel Res.* 2015; 473: 509–520.

Gioe, TG. *Third American Joint Replacement Registry Annual Report on Hip and Knees Arthroplasty Data.* Rosemont, IL: American Joint Replacement Registry, 2016.

Nebergall AK, Rolfson O, Rubash HE, Malchau H, Troelsen A, Greene ME. Stable fixation of a cementless, proximally coated, double wedged, double tapered femoral stem in total hip arthroplasty: A 5-year radiostereometric analysis. *J Arthroplasty.* 2016; 31(6): 1267–1274.

Nebergall AK, Troelsen A, Rubash HE, Malchau H, Rolfson O, Greene ME. Five-year experience of vitamin E-diffused highly cross-linked polyethylene wear in total hip arthroplasty assessed by radiostereometric analysis. *J Arthroplasty.* 2016; 31(6): 1251–1255.

ACKNOWLEDGMENTS

Central credit for creating my enthusiasm to write this story goes to my son, Jonathan. Jon had to overcome some well-established resistances. During my entire career I steadfastly declined nearly all urgings to write a book, and even resisted requests to contribute chapters to books, to the fullest extent possible. The underlying reason is because writing chapters in books takes time away from my primary commitments—namely, caring for patients and working in my lab. It was only through countless kind and considerate (and repeated) hints, suggestions, and reinforcement of the "need" that Jon broke down my lifetime resistance successfully.

Looking back on the whole process, Jon had an unknown ally from my past, for I had given the Presidential Guest Address at the meeting of the Hip Society in 2003, an address with a title similar to the subtitle of this book: "The Conquest of a Worldwide Disease." That article was published in 2004.* While that work had been based solidly on our research, it was, at that time, a prediction rather than a realization. I expressed the hope, the expectation, of conquering this disease, but the entire process of creating the rich and broadly based *proof* in patients that our ideas had merit was yet to come.

Once my mind was bent to the task, the first real step forward was generated by Elizabeth Law, daughter of Warren and Betty Law, who were longtime close friends in Belmont, Massachusetts. Elizabeth is a professional editor working in New York, albeit specializing in children's books. Her magic influence on me grew out of the reassurance that she would help guide me into the strange territories of both the arduous task of the actual writing and then exploring the "publishing jungle." Without her enthusiastic advice, the process would have stalled, again, at that threshold.

Through the advice of Elizabeth, I engaged a creative, smart, and effective writer—the accomplished Donna Beech—to facilitate my transition from 55 years of writing scientific articles into the challenging sphere of storytelling, creating an interesting and attractive story. Scientific writing, perforce, made me adhere to a rigid and constraining style that is the exact opposite of the engaging and enticing forms necessary to elicit interest in the general reading public. The stilted form of medical writing, largely dictated by Isaac Newton during the 17th century, follows a rigid format, excludes extraneous but enticing material, and is always under pressure to explain the situation in the least number of words. Moreover, since the mid 20th century, an abstract is required, which is placed ahead of the article. Thus, if a mystery novel were written in the style of a scientific article, the abstract would acknowledge in its last sentence that it was the maid who carried out the murder! It was Donna who had the complex task to overcome my 55 years of scientific writing.

Aid in navigating the daunting, multifaceted, and rapidly changing face of book publishing came from several wonderful sources in addition to Elizabeth Law, Donna Beech, and Anar Nanji, an Ismaili friend who was also engaged in a parallel pursuit.

Within the remarkable cohort of residents at the senior community where I now reside—Brookhaven at Lexington, Massachusetts—is a large subset of remarkable people who have provided me with extensive and unique advice concerning the single most critical aspect of publishing a book: getting it published. They range from former CEOs of publishing companies, to experienced editors, to successful (and unsuccessful) authors. Others were invaluable sounding boards and esteemed critics. They include Carol Howell, Jack Horner, Betty Law, Margo Lindsey, Joan Keenan, Jane Martin, Dick McAdoo, Michael Scott-Morton, and, outside Brookhaven, my brother, Jack Harris.

But the key aid, which proved to be the single most valuable, came from a close friend who had already made the successful transition from superb scientific writing to writing for the general public: Edward O. Wilson. In addition to being a university professor at Harvard, he holds two Pulitzer Prizes for his extraordinary efforts to educate and lead the general public. He warmly encouraged my efforts and climaxed that support by writing the Foreword to this book.

My editors at Oxford University Press, Rebecca Suzan, Emily Perry, and Tiffany Lu, have been both insightful and creative in the process of bringing this volume to press. And clearly, without the infinite patience of Anne Goodrich, who has tirelessly retyped draft after draft while chasing reference materials covering decades of time, nothing would have evolved.

*Harris WH. Conquest of a worldwide human disease: Particle-induced periprosthetic osteolysis. *Clin Orthop.* 2004; 429: 39–42.

ABOUT THE AUTHOR

William H. Harris

It was an inauspicious beginning. The simple survival of a tiny, fragile premature baby, weighing only three pounds, was unusual in 1927.

Most of those who did survive became blind because of the mistaken belief at the time that preemies should be immediately rushed into an environment with 100% oxygen. Not until 1954 did pediatricians realize this practice caused overdeveloped blood vessels in the eyes and permanent damage to the retina. Thankfully, Harris' father, a general practitioner with fearless determination, took his infant son home, away from the incubator and from the hospital, and saved his sight.

At the same time, the childbirth nearly killed his 29-year-old mother. Left with the scars from severe rheumatic heart disease, she came very close to death from congestive heart failure that day.

Yet Fortune smiled on the three-pound boy. He was born into a family with a strong medical foundation. Both his father and grandfather were physicians. In years to come, his brother and his nephew would become physicians, and his daughter would become a midwife.

In 1947, Harris graduated from Haverford College at the age of 19 with high honors in chemistry, as a member of Phi Beta Kappa. In 1951, he received his doctor of medicine degree from University of Pennsylvania as a member of Alpha Omega Alpha, the medical school honorary fraternity. After an internship and general surgical training at the Hospital of the University of Pennsylvania, Dr. Harris did his orthopaedic training in the Harvard Program at the Children's Hospital of Boston and the Massachusetts General Hospital. He pursued further education in orthopaedic research at the Oak Ridge Institute of Nuclear Studies and The Royal National Orthopaedic Hospital, London, England. Haverford College granted him a DSc degree in 2000.

In 1959, Dr. Harris was chief resident in orthopaedic surgery at the Massachusetts General Hospital, and he joined the staff in 1960. By 1974, he was chief of the arthroplasty unit and remained so until 2004. In 1975, he became a clinical professor of orthopaedic surgery and in 1997 he became the Alan Gerry clinical professor of orthopaedic surgery at Harvard Medical School.

During his 57-year career in orthopaedic surgery, Dr. Harris has consistently integrated the art and craft of musculoskeletal surgery with a deep commitment to the improvement of the science of the field.

The Harris Orthopaedic Laboratory at the Massachusetts General Hospital was founded in 1969 and directed by him until 2004.

As discussed in this book, Dr. Harris played an important role in unraveling the mysteries of an entirely novel disease—periprosthetic osteolysis—initiating the first steps pointing to its molecular biology, establishing the mechanism of the polyethylene wear, and finally developing the highly crosslinked polyethylene that has virtually eliminated this disease in metal-on-polyethylene total hip replacements worldwide. More than six million people are walking around now on this material, which made these implants both stable and resistant to that devastating disease.

Dr. Harris is also known for performing the world's first total hip replacement in a patient with a total developmental dislocation of the hip, and for creating the first effective, cement-free acetabular component. His work profoundly reduced fatal pulmonary emboli, improved implant design, innovated surgical techniques, produced registry follow-up studies, and promoted materials research. He has also made major contributions to the evaluation and quantification of results of hip surgery, allowing more precise assessments of proposed improvement in designs, materials, and techniques to enable more accurate quantification of the vital distinction between change and progress.

His investigations contributed to new understandings in skeletal metabolism, to quantification of the pressure in articular cartilage in vivo in the human acetabulum, and to the field of human limb replantation. Among other important concepts, he contributed strongly to the new and critical understanding that most osteoarthritis of the hip is caused by developmental abnormalities, not by a cartilage deficiency.

These achievements in his career as a scientist in the laboratory have been matched by his extensive clinical practice. He is a skilled surgeon with not only the lowest sepsis rate of his era, but also the lowest mortality rate of his era for total hip replacement surgery.

Dr. Harris has been honored with three Kappa Delta Awards, the highest award in North America for orthopaedic research. As of this writing, he is the only American to receive the Lifetime Achievement Award from the Muller Foundation, and he was the first Lifetime Achievement Award recipient of the International

Hip Society. The Hip Society has given him an unprecedented 10 research awards and chose him as the first surgeon to receive their Lifetime Achievement Award. He is the author of 523 refereed publications and 51 chapters of books.

In their 2013 nomination letters of Dr. Harris for the Lasker Award, often known as the American Nobel Prize, many leading physicians put his work in context. Dr. Thomas P. Sculco, Chairman of Orthopaedic Surgery, Weill Cornell Medical College, said frankly, "I can think of no other orthopaedic surgeon who has contributed to the improvement of our patients' lives as much as Dr. William Harris."

In addition to the important breakthroughs he has made as a medical scientist and as a clinician, Dr. Jorge O. Galante, MD, Rush University, observed that Dr. Harris will also leave a lasting legacy of gifted disciples who will make numerous research and clinical contributions to orthopaedic surgery.

For Dr. Henrik Malchau, a professor at Harvard Medical School and codirector of his eponymous Harris Orthopaedic Laboratory at the Massachusetts General Hospital, Dr. Harris is a highly respected surgeon and researcher, who is truly "a pioneer of modern-day hip surgical techniques and practices."

INDEX